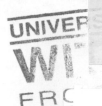

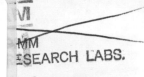
REVIEW COPY
We would appreciate your sending two copies of your review.

COVALENTLY MODIFIED ANTIGENS AND ANTIBODIES
IN DIAGNOSIS AND THERAPY
(Targeted Diagnosis and Therapy Series/2)

Edited by: Gerard A. Quash and John D. Rodwell

Published: 1989
248 pages, bound, illustrated

$ 99.75 (U.S. and Canada)
$119.50 (All other countries)
(Prices subject to change without notice.)

marcel dekker, inc.
270 MADISON AVENUE • NEW YORK, NY 10016 • 212–696–9000

Covalently Modified Antigens and Antibodies in Diagnosis and Therapy

Targeted Diagnosis and Therapy

Editor

John D. Rodwell
Vice President, Research and Development
CYTOGEN Corporation
Princeton, New Jersey

1. Antibody-Mediated Delivery Systems, *edited by John D. Rodwell*

2. Covalently Modified Antigens and Antibodies in Diagnosis and Therapy, *edited by Gerard A. Quash and John D. Rodwell*

3. Targeted Therapeutic Systems, *edited by Praveen Tyle and Bhanu P. Ram*

Covalently Modified Antigens and Antibodies in Diagnosis and Therapy

edited by

Gerard A. Quash
INSERM
Lyon, France

John D. Rodwell
CYTOGEN Corporation
Princeton, New Jersey

Marcel Dekker, Inc.   **New York • Basel**

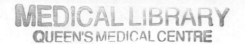
ISBN 0-8247-8107-4

This book is printed on acid-free paper.

MARCEL DEKKER, INC.
270 Madison Avenue, New York, New York 10016

Current printing (last digit):
10 9 8 7 6 5 4 3 2 1

PRINTED IN THE UNITED STATES OF AMERICA

Preface

Since the development by Kohler and Milstein of monoclonal antibodies, their use as finely tuned investigative tools has become more and more widespread. Associated with this, an abundance of markers has been linked to these unique immunoglobulins for both diagnostic and therapeutic applications. This volume evolved as a result of the symposium Covalently Modified Antigens and Antibodies in Diagnosis and Therapy cosponsored by the Institut National de la Santé et de la Recherche Medicale (INSERM) and CYTOGEN Corporation held in Lyon, France, in June, 1987. It was clear to lecturers and participants at this symposium that the science presented in plenary sessions, minisymposia and certain poster presentations should be enlarged upon and developed into a volume for the Targeted Diagnosis and Therapy series.

The effort has yielded an eclectic work that covers a lot of ground. Topics begin with a survey of the use of antibodies, vaccines, and anti-idiotypes in tumor therapy. Then, a variety of immunoconjugates for diagnosis and therapy in which the antibodies are coupled to a range of proteins, chemotherapeutic agents, and isotopes is discussed. Finally, a series of interesting systems in which antibodies (and/or antigens) are used in in vitro diagnostic or therapeutic procedures is explored. It is hoped that the reader will find this volume informative with respect to the variety of applications and approaches to immunodiagnosis and therapy.

As with any such work, the editors have many to thank. Mlle Aline Mary, Ms. Carol Peevey, and Ms. Joan Greenjak were invaluable in helping us solicit and edit manuscripts. Also, the staff at Marcel Dekker, Inc. assisted with a high degree of professionalism. We thank you all.

Gerard A. Quash
John D. Rodwell

Contents

Preface   iii

Contributors   vii

1. Karl Erik Hellström and Ingegerd Hellström   Immunological Approaches to Tumor Therapy: Monoclonal Antibodies, Tumor Vaccines, and Anti-Idiotypes   1

2. Pierre Carayon, Pierre Casellas, and F. K. Jansen   Biochemical Engineering of Immunotoxins for Ex Vivo Bone Marrow Transplantation and In Vivo Leukemia Treatment   41

3. Robert W. Baldwin and Vera S. Byers   Monoclonal Antibody 791T/36 Immunoconjugates for Cancer Treatment   53

v

4. Geoffrey A. Pietersz, Mark J. Smyth, Jerry Kannellos, Zita Cunningham, and Ian F. C. McKenzie — Preclinical Studies with Immuno-conjugates 73

5. Vernon L. Alvarez, A. Dwight Lopes, John D. Rodwell, and Thomas J. McKearn — Radioimmunoscintigraphy and Radioimmunotherapy in Nude Mice Models: Studies with Site-Specifically Modified Monoclonal Antibodies 99

6. Yoram Reiter and Zvi Fishelson — Killing of Human Tumor Cells by Antibody C3b Conjugates and Human Complement 119

7. Valérie Combaret, M. C. Favrot, and T. Philip — Marrow Purging for Autologous Bone Marrow Transplantation 137

8. Gerard A. Quash, Vincent Thomas, Georges Ogier, Said El Alaoui, Jean-Guy Delcros, Huguette Ripoll, Anne-Marie Roch, Richard Gilbert, Jean-Pierre Ripoll, and Stephane Legastelois — Diagnostic and Therapeutic Proced-ures with Haptens and Glycoproteins (Antigens and Antibodies) Coupled Covalently by Specific Sites to Insoluble Supports 155

9. Susan Y. Tseng, J. William Freytag, and Alan R. Craig — A Highly Sensitive EIA Utilizing Co-valent Conjugate of a Polymerized Enzyme and an Antibody 187

10. H. Phillip Lau, Robin Resch Charlton, Esther K. Yang, and Warren K. Miller — Immobilization of Antigens and Antibodies on Chromium Dioxide Magnetic Particles for Use in Immunodiagnostic Assays 201

11. Veronique Annaix, Abdelha-mid Bouali, and Jean-Marcel Senet — Use of Coated Latex Particles for Identification and Localization of *Candida albicans* Cell Surface Re-ceptors and for Detection of Related Circulating Antigens and/or Anti-bodies in Patient Sera and Urine 217

Index   231

Contributors

VERNON L. ALVAREZ, Ph.D. Director, Department of Chemical Research, CYTOGEN Corporation, Princeton, New Jersey

VERONIQUE ANNAIX UFR des Sciences Medicales et Pharmaceutiques-Section Pharmacie, Laboratoire d'Immunologie-Parasitologie-Mycologie, Angers, France

ROBERT W. BALDWIN, Ph.D. Professor, Director of Cancer Research Campaign Laboratories, University of Nottingham, Nottingham, England

ABDELHAMID BOUALI, Ph.D. UFR des Sciences Medicales et Pharmaceutiques-Section Pharmacie, Angers, France

VERA S. BYERS, M.D., Ph.D. Director, Clinical Investigations, Department of Clinical Research, XOMA Corporation, Berkeley, California

PIERRE CARAYON Ingenieur Biologiste, Head of the Laboratory of Cytofluorimetry, Immunology Department, Sanofi Recherche, Montpellier, France

PIERRE CASELLAS, Ph.D. Leader, Immunopharmacology Department, Sanofi Rechereche, Montpellier, France

ROBIN R. CHARLTON, Ph.D. Research Biochemist, Medical Products Department, E. I. duPont de Nemours & Co. Inc., Glasgow Research Laboratory, Wilmington, Delaware

VALERIE COMBARET Attaché de Recherche, Bone Marrow Transplant Unit, Centre Léon Berard, Lyon, France

ALAN R. CRAIG Senior Research Chemist, Medical Products Department, E. I. du Pont de Nemours & Co., Inc., Wilmington, Delaware

ZITA CUNNINGHAM Research Centre for Cancer and Transplantation, University of Melbourne, Victoria, Australia

JEAN-GUY DELCROS Unité de Virologie—INSERM, Lyon, France

SAID EL ALAOUI, Unité de Virologie—INSERM, Lyon, France

M. C. FAVROT Centre Léon Berard, Lyon, France

ZVI FISHELSON, Ph.D. Senior Scientist, Department of Chemical Immunology, The Weizmann Institute of Science, Rehovot, Israel

J. WILLIAM FREYTAG Research Manager, Medical Products Department, E. I. du Pont de Nemours & Co., Inc., Wilmington, Delaware

RICHARD GIBERT Ministère de la Santé, Départment d'étude des Maladies Virales, Laboratoire National de la Santé, Lyon, France

INGEGERD HELLSTRÖM Vice President, Department of Molecular Sciences, ONCOGEN, and Professor, Department of Microbiology, University of Washington Medical School, Seattle, Washington

KARL ERIK HELLSTRÖM Vice President, Department of Immunotherapy, ONCOGEN, and Professor, Department of Pathology, University of Washington Medical School, Seattle, Washington

F. K. JANSEN Sanofi Recherche, Montpellier, France

JERRY KANELLOS Research Centre for Cancer and Transplantation, University of Melbourne, Victoria, Australia

H. PHILLIP LAU, Ph.D. Senior Research Chemist, Medical Products Department, E. I. du Pont de Nemours Co., Inc., Glasgow Research Laboratory, Wilmington, Delaware

STEPHANE LEGASTELOIS Unité de Virologie-INSERM, Lyon, France

A. DWIGHT LOPES, VMD Group Leader, Department of Antibody Evaluation, CYTOGEN Corporation, Princeton, New Jersey

THOMAS J. McKEARN, M.D. Ph.D. Senior Vice President, Scientific Affairs, CYTOGEN Corporation, Princeton, New Jersey

IAN F. C. McKENZIE, M.D., Ph.D. Director Research Centre for Cancer and Transplantation, and Professor, Department of Pathology, University of Melbourne, Parkville, Victoria, Australia

WARREN K. MILLER, B.S. Development Associate, Medical Products Department, E. I. du Pont de Nemours & Co., Inc., Glasgow Research Laboratory, Wilmington, Delaware

GEORGES OGIER Unité de Virologie–INSERM, Lyon, France

T. PHILIP Centre Leon Berard, Lyon France

GEOFFREY A. PIETERSZ, Ph.D. Department of Pathology, Research Centre for Cancer and Transplantation, University of Melbourne, Parkville, Victoria, Australia

GERARD A. QUASH, Ph.D. Unité de Virologie–INSERM, Lyon, France

YORAM REITER, M.Sc. Research Student for Ph.D., Department of Chemical Immunology, The Weizmann Institute of Science, Rehovot, Israel

HUGUETTE RIPOLL Unité de Virologie–INSERM, Lyon, France

JEAN-PIERRE RIPOLL Hôpital Cardiovasculaire et Pneumologique, Lyon, France

RAYMOND ROBERT UFR des Sciences Médicales et Pharmaceutiques, Section Pharmacie, Laboratoire d'Immunology-Parasitologie-Micologie, Angers, France

ANNE-MARIE ROCH Unité de Virologie–INSERM, Lyon, France

JOHN D. RODWELL, Ph.D. Vice President, Research and Development, CYTOGEN Corporation, Princeton, New Jersey

JEAN MARCEL SENET UFR des Sciences Médicales et Pharmaceutiques-Section Pharmacie, Laboratoire d'Immunologie-Mycologie-Parasitologie, Angers, France

MARK J. SMYTH, Ph.D. Department of Pathology, Research Centre for Cancer and Transplantation, University of Melbourne, Parkville, Victoria, Australia

FRANK P. STUART, M.D. Professor, Department of Surgery, University of Chicago, Chicago, Illinois

VINCENT THOMAS Unité de Virologie—INSERM, Lyon, France

GUY TRONCHIN UFR des Sciences Médicales et Pharmaceutiques, Section Pharmacie, Laboratoire d'Immunologie-Parasitologie-Mycologie, Angers, France

SUSAN Y. TSENG Ph.D. Research Chemist, Medical Products Department, E. I. du Pont de Nemours & Co., Inc., Wilmington, Delaware

ESTHER K. YANG E. I. du Pont de Nemours Company, Inc., Glasgow Research Laboratory, Wilmington, Delaware

1

Immunological Approaches to Tumor Therapy
Monoclonal Antibodies, Tumor Vaccines, and Anti-Idiotypes

KARL ERIK HELLSTRÖM and INGEGERD HELLSTRÖM
Oncogen, Seattle, Washington
University of Washington Medical School, Seattle, Washington

I. INTRODUCTION

A. Preface

Cell surface molecules which are expressed preferentially by malignant cells can be used as "targets" for designing immunological approaches to cancer therapy, providing they are accessible to antibodies and/or lymphoid effector cells. The therapeutic target may be one which is naturally recognized as immunologically foreign by the cancer patient or which the patient can be made to recognize as such. It may also be a molecule which the patient is genetically incapable of reacting against (1), since such a molecule could be used to target to the tumor agents with antineoplastic activity, for example, an antibody conjugated to an anticancer drug. Thus, α-fetoprotein (2) and carcinoembryonic antigen (CEA) (3), which do not appear to be immunogenic in humans, are good candidates for tumor targeting (4).

We have for many years taken an interest in tumor markers which are recognized as antigenically foreign by the host, or which we believe could be recognized through the proper manipulation of the immune response. We focus on these markers with the hope of developing a "vaccine" for eliciting an immune response which could both mediate tumor destruction and have long-lasting activity against those neoplastic cells which escape more conventional forms of treatment. The type of vaccine we have in mind is for therapeutic use only, that is, for inducing in cancer patients an immune response which is clinically beneficial. For prophylactic use, antigens are needed that have a higher tumor specificity than is normally encountered in human neoplasms.

Many tumor antigens need to be evaluated before immunization to tumors will become a therapeutic reality and most of them will probably never prove useful for this purpose. Several antigens encountered during such an evaluation may, however, be suitable for the selective localization of anticancer agents to tumors, and would, therefore, still be important. In spite of our stated interest in tumor vaccines, we are working on both types of antigens.

We begin this chapter by placing the work to be covered in a historical perspective in the following section. Our chapter is based on a plenary lecture given at The International Conference on "Covalently Modified Antigens and Antibodies in Diagnosis and Therapy" in Lyon, France in June 1987; therefore, we have concentrated on reviewing investigations by our own group. Except when stated otherwise, the work has been done on human tumor antigens, and it has relied extensively on hybridoma technology.

B. Background

The first evidence that human cancer patients can form an immune response to tumors was obtained some 15 to 20 years ago when it was demonstrated that their blood lymphocytes are often cytotoxic to cultivated cells from the patients' own autochthonous tumors and to other tumors of the same type (5–8). Furthermore, evidence was found that several different tumor-associated antigens are expressed in the same neoplasm (9), and that at least some of these are differentiation antigens common to neoplastic cells and cells from certain fetal tissues (10). At about the same time, it was reported that sera from cancer patients contain antibodies both to antigens unique to a patient's own neoplasm (11) and to antigens shared by many tumors of the same type (5,12).

The presence of an immune response in cancer patients to both individually unique and shared tumor antigens has been confirmed in well-controlled serological studies (13-15). It has also been confirmed that many cancer patients have a lymphocyte-mediated cytolytic reactivity to the individually unique antigens (16,17). The evidence that there are cell-mediated responses to tumor-associated differentiation antigens has been less well accepted, particularly with respect to those responses which can cause tumor cell destruction in vitro (18). Nevertheless, the initial observation of lymphocyte-mediated cytolytic responses toward shared tumor antigens has been upheld in studies on both human (19–22) and animal (23,24) neoplasms. Furthermore, data supporting the view that lymphocytes from cancer patients react to shared, tumor-type-related antigens have come from many investigations with techniques measuring either leuko-cyte migration inhibition or leukocyte adherence inhibition (see, e.g., 25–28).

Although the findings referenced indicate that cancer patients often react immunologically to several different tumor antigens, this reactivity does not ap-pear to be very effective in limiting the growth of their tumors. At least part of the lack of efficacy can be attributed to an activation of suppressor cells (29–33), often associated with the presence of circulating suppressor ("blocking") factors (34–37). Consequently, therapeutic procedures deserve to be considered which aim at decreasing the suppressor activity (30–33). Alternatively, one may supply tumor-reactive lymphocytes that have reached a level of activation at which they are insensitive to suppression (37). Treatment with lymphokine-activated killer (LAK) cells (38), or interleukin-2- (IL-2) stimulated, tumor-infiltrating lymphocytes (39) may be viewed in this context.

Progress toward some form of therapeutic vaccination necessitates knowledge as to which antigens can induce an immune response in humans and how this response is regulated. Hybridoma technology (40) provides an excellent means of learning about various tumor antigens, because it both allows an in-depth investigation of their specificity and molecular nature and makes available ade-quate amounts of monoclonal antibodies (MAb) for in vivo testing against tumors. Furthermore, there is recent evidence that some patients who have re-ceived MAb to tumor-associated differentiation antigens have a favorable clinical response (41–43), and it has been suggested that a key component in this re-sponse is mediated by an immune reaction induced in the host (44). If the latter proves to be the case, the results obtained through the clinical testing of anti-tumor MAb should contribute to our understanding of regulation of tumor im-munity and help toward developing therapeutic tumor vaccines.

II. MELANOMA ANTIGEN p97

One of the best characterized human tumor antigens is a melanoma-associated cell surface glycoprotein called p97. Much of what has been learned about p97 can be used as a blueprint for approaches to study other tumor antigens, includ-ing those which are expressed on carcinomas, sarcomas, and lymphomas.

A. Specificity

p97 (45) was identified by using a mouse MAb, 4.1, which immunoprecipitates a glycoprotein with a molecular weight similar to that of rabbit phosphorylase b (97,400). It was found to be present in melanoma cells cultivated in vitro as well as in biopsies of melanoma. An antigen subsequently described by Dippold et al. and called gp95 (46), has proved to be identical to p97 (47), as has an antigen described by Khosravi et al. (48).

Several antibodies have been obtained which between themselves identify five different epitopes of p97 (46–49). Using pairs of antibodies to different epitopes of p97, a double-determinant immunoassay (DDIA) was developed (50). This assay, which is a variant of the classical immunoradiometric assay, is reliable for measuring p97 both on cells and in soluble form, and can detect less than 100 p97 molecules per cell. Employing DDIA for studies on a large variety of neoplastic and normal tissues, it became clear that most melanomas express more p97 than other tumors or various normal tissues (47,49). It also became apparent, however, that small amounts of p97 are expressed on normal cells from the adult host and that some normal fetal cells (e.g., from the intestinal epithelium) have relatively large amounts of the antigen (51). Most melanomas express 50,000–500,000 molecules of p97 per cell, as compared to about 300–8000 molecules per cell in normal tissues, the highest being detected in smooth muscle (47,50). Bone marrow stem cells have not been affected by anti-p97 MAb, when tested alone or in the presence of rabbit complement with assays measuring colony formation of four different types of stem cells (B. Torok-Storb et al., 1980).

The initial studies on p97 provided one of the first demonstrations that the specificity of a typical, MAb-defined human tumor antigen is relative rather than absolute. Subsequent work has found this to be true for other tumor-associated antigens that have been defined by mouse or human MAb, in all cases where it has so far been carefully examined (52,53).

B. Molecular Nature

p97 is a phosphorylated sialoglycoprotein (47). A partial N-terminal amino acid sequence showed that it is structurally related to transferrin (53). Like transferrin, p97 can bind iron (54). Furthermore, the genes for both p97 and transferrin are located within the chromosomal region 3q21–3q29, as is the transferrin receptor gene, the product of which is not structurally related to p97 or transferrin (55,56).

A cDNA clone encoding p97 was isolated (57), followed by genomic cloning of p97 and sequencing of the entire gene (58). The DNA sequencing data confirmed p97's substantial homology with transferrin, and they also showed that p97, as opposed to transferrin, has a small hydrophobic segment which is presumed to be a membrane-anchoring domain. Close homologues to the p97 gene have been identified in other species, including mice, birds, fishes, and tunicates (59).

Mouse MAb to human p97 do not cross-react with the mouse analogue of the antigen (59). Cultivated fibroblasts and Epstein-Barr virus (EBV)-transformed lymphocytes from non-human primates, on the other hand, express human p97 at approximately the same level as the corresponding human tissues (around 5000 molecules per cell), according to studies with a DDIA using mouse MAb (Estin et al., 1987, unpublished observations).

C. Transfection of Mouse Melanomas with the p97 Gene

In order to establish an animal model, the p97 gene has been transfected into mouse melanoma lines which then express the human form of p97 (60). When cells from the B16 mouse melanoma were transfected, no p97 was detected at the cell surface, while large amounts of antigen were released to the culture medium; such medium thus provides a good source of soluble p97 for purification. Transfection of the K1735-M2 melanoma of C3H/HeN origin did (61), on the other hand, induce the expression of p97 at the cell surface (60). Three transfected cell lines, A, B, and E, were obtained which express, on the average, between 2×10^5 and 10^6 molecules of p97 per cell, while the parental K1735-M2 melanoma has no detectable p97. The highest expressing line, A, does not form tumors when transplanted into syngeneic C3H/HeN mice. Lines B and E do, however, form lung metastases following intravenous inoculation and can also grow subcutaneously. They thus provide useful modules for various forms of therapy with the human p97 antigen as the target. The failure of the A line to form tumors in conventional mice is probably due to the strong immunogenicity of the p97 antigen, since this cell line can grow in nude mice (60).

D. In Vivo Localization of Anti-p97 MAb to Tumor

Studies in nude mice transplanted with p97 positive human melanomas showed that an intravenously injected anti-p97 antibody (MAb 96.5) localizes selectively to the tumors, as do Fab fragments prepared from the MAb (62). Two types of investigations in humans subsequently followed, using radiolabeled and unlabeled antibodies, respectively, and will now be discussed.

Several studies show that ^{131}I-labeled anti-p97 MAb (96.5) or its Fab fragments can localize better than control MAb or Fab to metastatic melanoma (62–66). Furthermore, the anti-p97 MAb or Fab localized to a greater extent in tumors than in normal tissues, while there was no such difference for the control MAb (or Fab). It became evident that Fab fragments localize more quickly to tumors than do whole MAb, accumulate less in normal tissues, and are less prone to induce an antibody response to mouse immunoglobulin. This implies that they are likely to be better for diagnostic imaging (64), a conclusion also reached by others (67).

That uptake of anti-p97 MAb (Fab) in tumor has immunological specificity was demonstrated by pair-labeling experiments with p97-specific and control MAb. Consecutive nuclear "imaging" of the same patient with both specific and control MAb revealed that only the specific MAb localized preferentially to the tumor (65). Cutaneous metastases, as well as visceral lesions could be identified (65). Using Fab fragments of anti-p97 antibodies, approximately 80% of all clinically detectable tumor nodules with a mean diameter of at least 10 mm were observed. It may be possible to obtain better resolution by labeling the Fab with ^{123}I or ^{99}mTc rather than ^{131}I (64), since the emission of gamma rays from these isotopes better fit the existing equipment in nuclear medicine laboratories.

Multicenter prospective studies with several different antimelanoma MAb are now needed to determine to what extent diagnostic imaging with labeled MAb and Fab fragments could contribute to the clinic. At least one study of this type has been done on a large number of melanoma patients and indicates that diagnostic imaging is informative in their clinical handling (68). The chapter by Mach in this volume concerns similar issues, but investigated patients with colorectal carcinoma.

Goodman et al. (69) reported that unlabeled MAb can be given safely to human patients with melanoma, and that it binds to tumor cells in vivo. The degree of accumulation of the injected MAb in tumor was assayed by immuno-histology on frozen sections of metastatic nodules which were removed at various time points after MAb infusion. MAb 96.5 (47) was the anti-p97 antibody used. This is an IgG2a that appears to have no antitumor activity when assayed in vitro or in nude mice (70). Most of the patients received MAb 96.5 together with another MAb, 48.7, which is an IgG1 specific for a melanoma-associated proteoglycan antigen (71). The largest MAb dose was 440 mg per patient and was administered over a 7-day period. The half life for the injected MAb in the circulation was approximately 30 h, and a peak serum antibody concentration of 60 μg/ml was obtained. Both MAb were found to localize to metastases and bound uniformly to neoplastic cells throughout the tumors as long as a sufficient dose was given. This dose was approximately >200 mg per patient for the MAb used. Within 2 to 4 weeks after MAb infusion, human anti-bodies to mouse immunoglobulin were detected in patient sera. In at least one case, they were found to be directed to idiotypic determinants (69).

The studies by the Larson and Goodman groups were of significance because they indicated that the p97 antigen is a good target for tumor therapy by being expressed on tumors growing in vivo and accessible to localization by MAb and Fab fragments.

E. Therapeutic Approaches Relating to p97

Several different therapeutic possibilities for anti-p97 MAb have been suggested by published work, including: Mouse MAb to p97 are cytolytic to p97-

positive tumor cells in t
synergistic effect when M
(72). Although no cytoly
been observed, it may be p
utilize the fact that MAb ca
Anti-p97 MAb conjugated w
ing $\geq 10,000$ molecules of p$^{\searrow}$
vindesine, cytotoxic activity o
of the antigen has been observe
therapeutically (66; also see belc
(75), as well as a p97-specific vacc
response of possible therapeutic va.

III. VARIOUS OTHER HUMAN TUN

As pointed out in the Introduction, hum
unique and shared antigens, with some of
expressed most strongly in tumors of the s.
many antigens which are present inside the c
are useful markers for immunohistological diag
been of primary interest as therapeutic targets, s.
lieved that they are more accessible to antibodies.
dismiss the possibility that some antigens which are
cellularly, could be good therapeutic targets. There is
to some intracellular antigens can be taken up by neopl.
there in very high concentrations for long periods of time
certain hormones (79). Furthermore, intracellular antigens
peptides resulting from "processing," be targets for cytolyti

A. Individually Unique Antigens

With a few exceptions (15), very little is known about the n
tumor antigens that are unique to individual patients, and th
tance of these antigens is limited by the need to "tailor-mak
product for each patient. Nevertheless, some of the most im
therapeutic work done with MAb has related to individually
which are present on B lymphomas in the form of idiotypic
In a patient with a B-cell lymphoma, the only normal cells c
infused MAb to the idiotype of the lymphoma would be the
which belong to the clone of cells from which the lymphon
hence, carry the respective idiotype at their surface. Conseq

t no damage to normal
) lymphocytes which

B lymphomas has re-
er the administration of
erapeutic failure has been
target idiotype (83,84),
tocol may be beneficial. For
radiolabeled with a radioiso-
cussed below, can also kill

hich are shared by human neoplasms
antigens which initially appeared to
nt also on normal cells, albeit at much
yzed (45,49,53).
of antigens that are truly tumor specific
tial therapeutic use of MAb. In most cases,
ted antigen is probably sufficient for targeting
shold level of antigen expression at the cell sur-
e cells are killed by conjugates between antibodies
.E) or destroyed by antibody-mediated cellular
-mediated cytotoxicity, or cytolytic T cells.
ong the first human tumors studied. In addition to the
iscussed), they expressed a proteoglycan (71,85) and sev-
46,85–88) and glycolipid (46,89,90) antigens. There is a
s which are expressed most strongly on carcinomas. These
cin identified on human breast, colon, and ovarian carcin-
3 (91), antigens demonstrated in colon carcinomas by anti-
10 (86), protein and glycolipid antigens of small cell (92)
–95) lung carcinomas, a carbohydrate antigen detected in
omas by MAb L6 (95), antigens expressed in kidney car-
ntigen shared by sarcomas and several carcinomas (97).
antigens have been detected in lymphomas, including
9), and Bp50 (100). Altogether, hundreds of MAb to
have been obtained over the past few years, and we make
them all here. Rather, we refer the reader to some recent

IV. THERAPEUTIC USERS OF ANTITUMOR
ANTIBODIES IN THE UNMODIFIED FORM

A. Antibodies with Antitumor Activity

A simple way of applying antitumor MAb clinically is to administer them in the unmodified form, using as the logical choices MAb which display antitumor activity in vitro and in nude mice. Antibodies to molecules which play key roles in tumor cell proliferation and/or invasiveness are of particular interest, because they may inhibit neoplastic growth, prevent tumor cells from metastasizing, and/or induce tumor cell differentiation. Some MAb that appear to prevent tumor cell invasion have been obtained (106,107).

Although most MAb to tumor antigens do not appear to have any antitumor activity by themselves, there are several MAb which mediate complement-dependent cytotoxicity (CDC) in the presence of human serum as a source of complement (70,108), or antibody-dependent cellular cytotoxicity (ADCC) together with either human NK cells (70,89,109,110) or macrophages (111,112). Antibodies that can kill human tumor cells when combined with complement from rabbits or guinea pigs, but not from humans, also exist (72) but are of less interest in this context.

The rationale for therapeutic use of MAb with ADCC and CDC is that such MAb often have antitumor activities in vivo as observed either in nude mice (see below) or in syngeneic mouse tumor models (113). Antibodies lacking ADCC and CDC activity in vitro, on the other hand, are commonly ineffective in vivo, unless used as carriers of antitumor agents. According to studies in a syngeneic mouse model, the ability of a MAb to mediate ADCC correlates with its antitumor activity in vivo, while there are MAb with CDC (but not ADCC) activity which lack in vivo efficacy (114); for this, however, complement which was not of mouse origin was used. It is not known whether the situation in humans will be similar, and we continue to take a great interest in IgG MAb with CDC activity in the presence of human complement because we believe that the ability of MAb to activate the host's complement may prove to be therapeutically beneficial: tumor cells may be killed, the blood supply to tumors may increase, thereby facilitating their uptake of drugs, etc.

Among mouse MAb, the IgG_2a and IgG_3 isotypes are most commonly associated with ADCC and CDC. For example, MAb MG-21 (IgG_3), which is specific for a melanoma-associated GD3 glycolipid, can mediate ADCC, lysing 50–100% of cultured, ^{51}Cr-labeled melanoma cells over a 4-h incubation period, and giving ADCC even at 0.1 $\mu g/ml$ (70). A concentration of 0.1 $\mu g/ml$ should be easy to achieve in tumor tissue following the intravenous administration of a few hundred milligrams of whole MAb (69).

The CDC data referred to with MG-21 could be confirmed with samples which were obtained directly from biopsies of metastatic melanoma and tested by a clonogenic assay. MG-21 concentrations of 10 μg/ml and the presence of human complement, produced close to 100% inhibition of colony formation (115). No differences have been detected by either the ^{51}Cr release or the clonogenic assay between the ability of serum from cancer patients and normal controls to serve as a source of complement (116).

The effector cells mediating ADCC, as measured by a 4-h ^{51}Cr release assay, have the characteristics of large granular lymphoid (LGL) cells and express the CD16 marker (108,110). They thus belong to the NK cell family. Monocytes and macrophages can also serve as effectors if they are incubated with the target cells for a period of 8–72 h (111,112). Patients with metastatic tumors often have depressed NK cell activity and a very low ability to mediate ADCC (110,116). It is important, therefore, that in vitro exposure of nonreactive lymphocytes to interferon or IL-2 can make them effective in mediating ADCC (110,116).

B. Studies in Nude Mice and Rats

Antibodies with ADCC and/or CDC activity have been injected into nude (athymic) mice or rats bearing human tumors in order to study the antitumor activities in vivo. One must realize, however, that such animal models are highly artificial. Normal mouse and rat cells entirely lack the target antigens (which is not the case in humans), and t cell-dependent immune responses to tumor antigens cannot be induced in athymic animals (while they can in humans).

Although inhibition of the outgrowth of xenografted tumors has been observed with several MAb given to nude mice (41,70,86,108,110), large tumors have generally not been rejected or even inhibited. It is interesting, therefore, that more encouraging data have recently been obtained in experiments with nude rats (Neuwelt et al., 1987, unpublished observations), which appear to have a more potent NK cell response than nude mice. Nude rats which had been transplanted with a human small cell lung carcinoma, LX1, both subcutaneously and in the brain, were injected intravenously with MAb L6 when they reached tumor diameter $\geq$ 10 mm and they were cachectic. In control animals tumors resulted in death within less than 2 weeks, however, 4 of 25 rats receiving MAb L6 underwent complete tumor regression and remained tumor free when the experiment was terminated more than 200 days later. Regression was never seen in untreated rats or in any of more than 100 rats given various other antitumor MAb.

Honsik et al. have stimulated human peripheral blood lymphocytes with IL-2 in vitro and then administered them together with antitumor MAb and IL-2 to nude mice transplanted with human tumors. In these experiments antitumor activity was observed also against established tumors (117). Therefore, combination therapies employing MAb and IL-2 seem attractive also in view of the evidence (discussed above) that the in vitro reactivity of NK cells is decreased in cancer patients and can be restored by exposure to IL-2.

C. Studies in Humans

Studies have been done in which patients with metastases from solid tumors have received up to several grams of MAb to shared tumor-associated antigens (41,42,118-120); clinical trials using MAb to clone-specific antigens on B lymphoma were discussed in a preceding section. Clinical responses have been shown, including a few complete and long-lasting remissions and several partial remissions. Although these responses are rare, they are probably too frequent to be attributed to random variation. They have been seen not only with skin metastases in melanoma, which are known to sometimes undergo spontaneous remission, but also in melanoma patients with visceral metastases. More important, they have been observed also with different carcinomas and the data have been obtained by several groups of investigators. MAb that have induced responses have been those that mediate ADCC and CDC in vitro and have some antitumor effect in nude mice. There is no clear-cut relationship between the dose of MAb injected and the clinical benefit, however. Responses have been observed in patients receiving as little as a few milligrams of MAb, which is likely to be too little to reach all the tumor cells. Clinical effects have been observed to occur after a lag time from 2 weeks to several months. Host immunity relating to the tumor is common in the form of antibodies to the idiotypes of the injected mouse MAb (44,69) and/or the presence of cytolytic T lymphocytes (121).

We speculate that the clinical responses observed were initiated by MAb destroying tumor cells and that this was followed by the presentation of tumor-associated differentiation antigens to the immune system in the form of complexes with mouse immunoglobulin. Most likely, immunological suppression occurs when lymphocytes are normally exposed to tumor-associated differentiation ("self") antigens. However, such antigens complexed with a foreign protein (mouse immunoglobulin) may induce immunological help rather than suppression. The immune response leading to clinical benefit may be the one that is induced to the particular antigen to which the MAb is directed, but it may also be one that is induced concomitantly but is specific for some other tumor antigen, which may either be shared or individually unique. It is unclear to what extent the clinical effects, when observed, are due to actual tumor destruction or are caused by changes which are induced in tumor cells and lead to either their suicide or differentiation toward normalcy.

V. CHIMERIC ANTIBODIES FOR TUMOR THERAPY

A. Problems with Mouse MAb

There are at least two problems inherent in using mouse MAb for the treatment of human tumors. First, they are recognized as foreign molecules, inducing an immune response to both framework and idiotypic determinants. Second, most mouse MAb are of isotypes which fail to mediate ADCC or CDC. As discussed in the preceding section, it must be realized, however, that the recognition of mouse MAb as foreign may not be entirely bad, because it may facilitate the induction of a potentially beneficial host response.

The induction of human antibodies to an injected mouse MAb can create difficulties in using such MAb for long-term treatment. Fab fragments have been found to be substantially less immunogenic than whole MAb (65,122,123). Therefore, one would expect an antibody which lacks the mouse Fc to have advantages for repeated use; human MAb or "chimeric" (mouse-human) MAb then come to mind. In order to convert a nonfunctional MAb to one with ADCC and/or CDC activity, one can use established techniques for isotype switching (124). It seems probable, however, that an antibody with the appropriate human Fc region might be better than any mouse MAb in mediating ADCC with human effector cells and CDC with human complement.

Although several human MAb to tumor antigens have been obtained (125–127), many do not appear to induce a B-cell response in cancer patients (128). It is important, therefore, that techniques have been developed by which chimeric antibodies can be made by splicing mouse genes coding for the variable region of the antibody molecule with human genes encoding the constant region (129,130). Such an approach has been used to prepare a variety of chimeric antibodies including some that are specific for tumor antigens (131–135).

B. Chimeric L6 and 2H7 Antibodies

We have conducted a collaborative study leading to the establishment and analyses of two different chimeric antibodies (134). One mouse MAb used is L6, which is specific for a carbohydrate antigen present on many different carcinomas and which mediates ADCC and CDC with human effector cells (70). The other mouse MAb, 2H7, is an IgG_2b which reacts with Bp35, a differentiation antigen of normal and neoplastic B cells, but lacks both ADCC and CDC activities (99). The chimeric antibodies were obtained by isolating cDNA clones for the heavy and light chains of the variable regions from the respective mouse hybridomas, and splicing those together with genes encoding the constant part of human IgG_1 (134,135). The primary reasons for choosing IgG_1 was that it is highly effective in mediating CDC and ADCC.

Chimeric L6 binds to antigen-positive cells with approximately the same affinity as mouse L6, and it does not bind to antigen-negative cells (134). While there is no difference between mouse and chimeric L6 with respect to CDC activity, the ADCC obtained with chimeric L6 was shown to be approximately 100 times greater than that with mouse L6. Thus, it was strong enough to lyse essentially 100% of antigen-positive tumor cells even at a concentration of 10 ng/ml. Additionally, there are significant ADCC with cells from a melanoma line, M-2669, which express a very low level of the L6-defined antigen and are not lysed by mouse L6 (134). Target cells not binding MAb L6, including cells from B and T lymphomas, were not affected.

The functional difference between chimeric and mouse antibodies was even more striking in studies with MAb 2H7. This is because mouse 2H7 does not give ADCC or CDC, while the chimeric 2H7 mediates both activities very effectively (135).

We conclude that chimeric antibodies deserve consideration as candidates for cancer therapy in anticipation of lesser immunogenicity in vivo, and because of their greater biological activity. Beyond using the chimeric antibodies as carriers of antitumor agents, the potent biological functions demonstrated in vitro makes it seem highly worthwhile to investigate their therapeutic effectiveness in the unmodified form.

It is likely, however, that chimeric (as well as entirely human) antibodies will induce anti-idiotypic responses, which may interfere with their repeated use. This may occur as easily as with mouse MAb, although it is possible that the presentation of an idiotype on a human framework may render it less immunogenic. If responses to idiotypic determinants will prevent long-term uses of the same MAb, it may prove necessary to establish a series of different MAb with the same specificity for antigen, since such MAb commonly display different idiotypes. For prolonged treatment of the same patient, some method for "tolerizing" the patient toward the injected immunoglobulin will, nevertheless, probably be needed (136).

The availability of cloned antibody genes may have further implications, which may prove to be very important. Thus it may be possible to combine antibody genes with genes coding for therapeutically desirable functions in order to develop new therapeutic agents. They may be in the form of molecules that have both the antibody's ability to bind to the target antigen and the ability to induce the differentiation of tumor cells into normal cells or to modulate lymphocyte responses, to give two examples.

VI. TARGETING OF RADIOACTIVE ISOTOPES

The fact that intravenously injected radiolabeled MAb (and fragments prepared from them) can localize with some selectivity to tumors suggests that a therapeutically effective radiation dose may be delivered by simply increasing the amount of radiolabel present on the injected MAb as well as the amount of MAb injected (65). Some provocative findings have been obtained by this approach. Carrasquillo et al. have reported one case where tumor growth was arrested and one case with partial tumor regression following the injection of ^{131}I-labeled

Fab fragments specific for melanoma-associated p97 or proteoglycan antigens (66). DeNardo et al. have observed tumor remissions in several leukemia patients given radiolabeled antibody (137). Work by Order et al. (who pioneered the use of radiolabeled antibodies for tumor therapy) has led to regressions in patients with Hodgkin's disease and hepatoma after injection of radiolabeled antibody to tumor-associated ferritin or alphafetoprotein (138–142).

The feasibility of localizing a therapeutic dose of radiation to tumor has thus been demonstrated. An advantage of this approach is that it may be possible to destroy tumor cells which, as a reflection of their heterogeneity (143–145), lack the antigen to which a given MAb is directed. This may be accomplished by using an isotope that emits beta particles, since they could be emitted from antibodies bound to antigen-positive tumor cells, penetrate a short distance through the tissue, and kill all the cells with which they come in contact.

For further discussions of this area, which is one of high therapeutic promise, we refer the reader to other contributions in this volume.

VII. IMMUNOCONJUGATES

Another use of antitumor MAb is in the form of immunoconjugates for the delivery of antitumor drugs and/or toxins to tumors. An advantage of using immunoconjugates is that one may selectively increase the amount of cytocidal/cytostatic agent localized to the tumor and hence decrease its sytemic toxicity. This may be therapeutically beneficial, even if the localization characteristics of the antibody would only allow the concentration of drug (toxin) to be two or three times greater in the tumor than in normal tissues. Judging from the experience gained by using radiolabeled antibodies, this degree of selectivity may be easily obtained and even exceeded (65), sometimes with a wide margin (78). An advantage of immunoconjugates over radiolabeled MAb is a logistic one, since it is much easier to treat patients with conjugates than to use high doses of radioactivity. There may also be less toxicity. Potential problems may be to obtain a conjugate which is sufficiently potent to kill the tumor and to devise a strategy for killing tumor antigen-negative cell variants. We (4) and others (146–148) have recently reviewed this area, which will, therefore, be dealt with only superficially here.

Immunoconjugates based on commonly used chemotherapeutic drugs come first to mind, as there is much experience using these drugs in the unconjugated form (4), which makes it relatively easy to establish whether a conjugate is any better than the free drug. One may also be able to use highly potent drugs which had to be excluded from systemic use because of toxicity, since effective conjugates may be prepared which have acceptable toxicity by being relatively

selective for the tumor. The use of immunotoxins (146,148,149) may be viewed
in that context, and it has been reported that immunotoxins between MAb and
ricin A chain have clinical activity in some melanoma patients (150), although
too few responses were seen to conclude that the conjugates were effective.

Because there are few, if any, antigens with absolute specificity for tumor,
one may often take advantage of the fact that a threshold level of antigen expression is needed before sufficient amounts of conjugate will bind to the cells
for killing to occur (as discussed previously). In many cases, there may be a
problem, however, to target to the tumor the amount of anticancer agent
needed to achieve a therapeutic result. The potency of the agent, the amount
that can be bound to each antibody molecule, the number of antibody molecules that can bind to each tumor cell, and the number of immunoconjugate
molecules that can be localized to each tumor cell in vivo, are all key factors.
A highly potent drug (or a toxin) may need to be chosen when only a few conjugate molecules will bind to the tumor cells in vivo. There may, however,
be some complications using highly toxic agents. While the expression of trace
levels of a tumor antigen on normal cells may be unimportant for a drug with
moderate potency, this needs to be taken seriously into account for a very
potent drug. One must also be aware that part of any injected immunoconjugate will be taken up in an antigen-nonspecific manner by normal tissues, particularly by the liver, spleen, kidney, and bladder (65). It becomes important
to obtain conjugates which remain bound to tumor for a substantially longer
time than they remain in blood or in normal tissues, as has been achieved with
some MAb (78).

Several immunoconjugates with drugs or toxins have been prepared and show
selective cytotoxicity on antigen-positive cells in vitro (4,75,76,148,149,151).
Some of these conjugates have been tested in nude mice carrying antigen-
positive human tumor xenografts (73,149) or in syngeneic animal models (148,
151), and have shown some efficacy. So far, however, there has been no con-
vincing demonstration that drug conjugates are effective in human cancer patients. Novel approaches may be needed, therefore, for increasing the level of
drug selectively delivered to the tumor. A conjugate allowing the release in the
tumor area of free drug which can diffuse into the tumor cells, appears more
attractive than one which has to be taken up by the cells. This is because the uptake of intact conjugates occurs at a very low level, except for a small number
of cases where an antibody bound to a surface antigen is internalized as commonly occurs by "capping" (152), akin to the mechanism responsible for antigenic modulation (153). Furthermore, tumors contain cells which do not express
a given antigen (92,93), which allows for the selection of antigen-negative variants. Although the use of MAb "cocktails" would help, it may not be sufficient
to solve this problem.

An attractive option would be to obtain a therapeutic agent which is not toxic until it comes in contact with the tumor, but once it localizes there produces a cytocidal compound as a result of either the selective release of a drug or its activation. A collaborative study between Drs. E. Lavie, L. Hill, K. Thor, and ourselves aims toward this goal (154,155). It is based on the evidence that the pH of tumor tissue is generally 0.5 to 1.0 units lower than that of normal tissues (156), and has led to the development of pH-sensitive conjugates between MAb L6 and the drug daunomycin, using established techniques (157). The conjugates bind selectively to cells expressing the antigen defined by MAb L6, they release free daunomycin at acid pH, and they localize to tumors when injected into nude mice (154,155). We do not yet know whether they have therapeutic activity in vivo.

Other approaches may involve the use of an enzyme which is present naturally at high levels within a tumor or which is localized to the tumor by an antibody. Such an enzyme could cause the release (or activation) of a cytocidal compound from a second agent which is given systemically and has low toxicity by itself. An advantage of using a conjugate for targeting an enzyme to tumor is that one may then give the second agent at a point of time when the conjugate is present at high levels in the tumor and at very low levels in various normal tissues including blood. As the second agent one may opt to use a conjugate with a MAb to a different tumor antigen, because this could increase the level of therapeutic selectivity (since two different tumor antigens then have to be recognized for a cytocidal event to happen). Another approach is to target an enzyme to the tumor and then given an inactive prodrug, which is converted to active anticancer drug at the tumor site (193). (Added in proof.)

Conjugates should also be considered which are capable of targeting immunomodulating agents, such as interferons, IL-2, endotoxins, or haptens to which a delayed-type hypersensitivity (DTH) reaction could be induced in the tumor area, as well as conjugates which may be able to induce tumor cell differentiation.

The use of bifunctional antibodies may be considered in this context. One antibody arm could then bind to tumor cells and the other could, for example, mediate a signal which would activate target cell killing by NK cells, as can mouse MAb 9.1 (158). A similar approach, using the appropriate MAb, may prove useful for activating cytolytic T cells or inhibiting the activity of suppressor T cells in the tumor area.

VIII. TUMOR VACCINES

A. General Approach

Active immunization is generally more effective than passive immunization in inducing resistance to microorganisms and in causing the rejection of transplanted neoplastic cells expressing tumor antigens. A rational therapeutic approach may thus be to develop immunogens (vaccines) for increasing the level of antitumor resistance in an antigen-specific way (8). This approach has strong merits, because active immunization is potentially more effective and long-lasting than the result of passively transferred MAb. Furthermore, vaccines are generally easy to administer and inexpensive. It must be realized, however, that a patient subjected to some form of tumor vaccination cannot be severely immunosuppressed, as is often the case late in the disease or when patients are undergoing chemotherapy.

When considering active immunotherapy of cancer, an important issue is the extent to which a tumor-associated differentiation antigen is viewed as "self" by the immune system. Those antigens which can induce an immune response in patients (22), and hence are recognized as foreign, appear to be the most logical candidates for vaccine development. However, except for a few cases, the molecular nature of these antigens is unknown (159), while there are many well-characterized antigens to choose from which have been defined by MAb. We have, therefore, taken an interest in the MAb-defined antigens, although very little is known about their immunogenicity in humans. We have done so under the assumption that some of these antigens, even if they are not naturally immunogenic in humans, can be made immunogenic by using the proper approach.

A patient with a progressively growing neoplasm is likely to have a large supply of antigen provided by the tumor. Immunization with unmodified antigen would thus not be expected to be very useful therapeutically, and may, at best, be employed to maintain antitumor resistance after the primary tumor has been removed. Activation of the immune system in a more powerful way is likely to be needed in cases where there is substantial metastatic spread. There are two types of vaccines that may fit this purpose: those that present tumor antigens to the immune system and those that present anti-idiotypic antibodies. The reason we take an interest also in the anti-idiotypic antibodies is that we believe, based on work in model systems (see below), that such antibodies might be able to favorably modify the immune response of the tumor-bearing host by inducing strong T-cell help or effectively decreasing suppressor cell activity.

B. Recombinant Live Virus Vaccines

When considering antigens as vaccines, we have chosen to work on recombinant live virus vaccines which are prepared by introducing the gene for a tumor antigen into the vaccinia virus genome (160). Vaccines of this type are attractive for at least two reasons: the tumor antigen is presented on macrophages and other cells, in close proximity to the host's own histocompatibility antigens, and it is "seen" by the immune system together with highly immunogenic vaccinia virus proteins which serve as excellent adjuvants (161).

Two studies using this recombinant vaccinia virus approach have been published. In one case, a vaccine was made containing an antigen of Friend virus-induced mouse leukemias (162), and in another case the antigen derived from polyoma virus-induced mouse tumors (163). Neither of these vaccines could be directly applied to humans, because the antigens in question do not have any human counterparts.

The availability of a cloned gene for a human tumor-associated differentiation antigen, p97, has allowed Estin et al. to develop a live, recombinant, vaccinia virus-based vaccine, vp97 (76). We shall discuss this work in some detail, since it may serve as a model for similar approaches to a variety of tumor-associated differentiation antigens.

Infection of cells with vp97 induces the expression of high levels of both p97 and vaccinia virus protein at their cell surface. When the vaccine is given to mice by scarification of the tail, high titers of anti-p97 antibodies are seen, and T cells from the immunized mice proliferate when exposed to either soluble p97 or mouse tumor cells expressing the p97 antigen (164). Furthermore, mice given vp97 develop delayed-type hypersensitivity (DTH) when challenged in the footpad with mouse tumor cells expressing p97 but not when challenged with p97-negative tumor cells. Although soluble p97 protein is as effective as vp97 in inducing both anti-p97 antibodies and a proliferative lymphocyte response, it does not induce DTH to p97.

Estin et al. have immunized C3H mice with vp97 and studied the effect on implanted syngeneic mouse melanomas that express p97 after transfection with the p97 gene (76). Mice immunized with vp97 by tail scarification developed resistance to transplants of syngeneic melanoma lines expressing p97 but not to the nontransfected, p97-negative parental line, and there was no resistance in mice immunized with vaccinia virus of the wild type (76). The antitumor activity was detected in vp97-immunized mice that were challenged with tumor cells subcutaneously, as well as in mice that were given tumor cells intravenously and subsequently developed lung metastases. Although mice immunized with soluble p97 had high titers of anti-p97 antibodies, they were not resistant to challenge with p97-positive tumor cells. This illustrates an advantage of the reccombinant virus vaccine over immunization with protein.

Clinical use of vp97 would primarily apply to patients with metastatic melanoma following "debulking" of their tumors, therefore, it is important to know whether immunization with vp97 can cause the rejection of mouse tumors growing either subcutaneously or in the lung. In the experiments done so far, immunization was started as early as two days after tumor transplantation. Antitumor activity was observed, both as a prolongation of time before the mice developed tumors of a certain size, and as a curative effect in some of the mice. The percentage of tumor-free survivors depended on what tumor line was used for the challenge. If line B was used where all the cells expressed p97 according to analysis with a fluorescence-activated cell sorter, 90 to 100% of long-term survivors were observed. If, on the other hand, line E was employed, which contained approximately 40% p97 negative cells, there were about 20% long-term survivors. The tumors that grew out in 80% of the mice primarily consisted of cells lacking p97. So far, therapeutic effects have unfortunately not been observed against large established tumors; the model system should lend itself very well to studying how this may be best achieved.

The fact that 20% long-term survivors were seen in mice challenged with the E line implies that the approximately 40% of p97-negative cells present within the tumor may have been killed as "bystanders" when the host's immune system rejected the p97-positive tumor cells. This may relate to the fact that tumor cells are sometimes killed at the site of a DTH reaction (165–167). This has important implications if a vaccine such as vp97 is to be used clinically, since tumors are heterogeneous with respect to antigen expression (144,145,149).

The data referred to show that an immune response to p97 can lead to tumor destruction under favorable circumstances, that is, when p97 is a foreign antigen as it is in mice, and the tumors are small. They give, however, no information as to whether an immune response to p97 can be induced in humans, whose normal tissues express trace amounts of p97.

As a step in this direction, experiments have been done in monkeys, *Macaca fascicularis*. Monkeys have a p97 homologue which, as far as it has been tested, is indistinguishable from the p97 of human cells. Antibodies to three different determinants of human p97 have been shown to bind to cultured normal cells from either man or monkey, with approximately 5000 molecules of p97 being detected at the cell surface in both cases. This is in sharp contrast to mouse cells to which mouse anti-p97 MAb do not bind at all. Two adult monkeys (Nos. 1 and 2) received vp97 by scarification, while a third monkey (No. 3) received wild-type vaccinia virus. Monkeys Nos. 1 and 2 developed anti-p97 antibodies and their lymphocytes proliferated in vitro when exposed to soluble p97. Furthermore, antibodies from both monkeys mediated ADCC on p97-positive tumor cells, and monkey No. 2 displayed DTH when challenged intradermally with p97. The control monkey (No. 3) neither made anti-p97 antibodies nor developed cellular immunity to p97. None of the monkeys showed any side effects associated with the vaccination, and autopsies performed 3 months after the immunizations showed no evidence of either macroscopic or microscopic tissue damage.

The fact that immunization with vp97 has antitumor activity in mice and induces humoral and cell-mediated immune responses to p97 in monkeys, suggests that such immunization might be clinically beneficial in human melanoma patients with p97-positive tumors. It is encouraging that DTH is part of the immune response induced, also in monkeys, in light of its apparent involvement in tumor rejection (165,168).

We speculate that vaccination with vp97 may cause the destruction of melanoma cells in human patients while sparing normal cells which express only trace amounts of p97 and are relatively resistant to killing by activated macrophages (as present at the site of a DTH). However, there are many questions which can only be answered by a clinical trial in humans. For example, will a vaccinated human patient form an immune response to p97 as did the monkeys? If so, will this response be powerful enough to kill both p97-positive melanoma cells and any p97-negative tumor cell variants? Will normal tissues be damaged? To what extent does a suppressor cell response occur when there is disseminated tumor, and will it prevent immunization against p97? If so, can this response be counteracted, allowing the treatment of disseminated tumors? What is the need for macrophages and other accessory cells in tumor rejection, and will this be a limiting factor? What is the role of cytolytic T cells and of antibodies mediating ADCC and CDC? Only some of these questions lend themselves to all studies on the mouse model.

There are other antigens that may be even better than p97 for the development of live recombinant viral vaccines. Antigens of papilloma virus, as expressed on many cervical carcinomas deserve to be considered, since these antigens may be more directly related to the cause of the neoplastic transformation (169). The risks for normal tissue damage may thus be less. Antigens of this type might possibly be candidates for development of prophylactic vaccines.

C. Anti-idiotypic Antibodies

Another approach for active tumor immunization is to use anti-idiotypic antibodies. Such antibodies have been employed as vaccines against bacteria, parasites, and viruses (170,171), whereby acting as "internal images" they have substituted for antigen. This has been particularly useful in cases where the antigens have been carbohydrates, which are difficult to obtain in sufficient amounts and of sufficient purity to use as immunogens. Anti-idiotypic antibodies have also been valuable in cases where one has a MAb to a microorganism but has not purified and characterized the target antigen to a sufficient extent to use it as an immunogen. We have reviewed the use of anti-idiotypic antibodies for tumor therapy (172–174) and thus will limit ourselves here to the following discussion.

Anti-idiotypic antibodies have been made relating to different tumor antigens, and antitumor effects have been observed in several animal systems. In some cases, the anti-idiotypic antibodies have related to individually unique, tumor-specific transplantation antigens of chemically induced mouse sarcomas (175,176). In other cases the antigens have either been encoded by a tumor virus (177), or they have been tumor-associated differentiation antigens like

those expressed in human neoplasms (178). For example, Nepom et al. (75) immunized rabbits with a MAb to p97 and obtained an anti-idiotypic poly-clonal serum which bound specifically to the immunizing MAb as well as to other MAb to the same p97 determinant. When injected into mice, this serum induced both DTH to p97 and antibodies capable of precipitating p97. Herlyn et al. obtained similar results with anti-idiotypic antibodies relating to an anti-gen of colorectal cancer (179). Koprowski et al. reported that human cancer patients responding favorably to therapy with unmodified mouse antibodies commonly develop anti-idiotypic antibodies (44). Their study suggests that anti-idiotypic antibodies relating to human tumor-associated differentiation antigens may indeed have therapeutic value in humans. However, direct proof of this point is still lacking.

Some of the more extensive animal studies on the therapeutic use of anti-idiotypic MAb have been done by Nelson et al., using two different anti-idio-typic MAb 4.72 and MAb 5.96 which relate to individually unique, tumor-specific transplantation antigens present on the chemically induced mouse sar-comas, MCA-1490 and MCA-1511 (176). Both DTH and, more important, the regression of small transplanted tumors were observed when MAb 4.72 or 5.96 was given to mice (175,176). These effects had antigen specificity as proven by parallel studies with two different sarcomas and the two anti-idio-typic MAb. Neither MAb 4.72 or MAb 5.96 bound to sarcoma cells. They did, however, bind to suppressor factors present in the sera of mice carrying the respective sarcomas. This binding had specificity for the antigen of the given tumor. Nelson et al. had previously established a T-T hybridoma by hybridiz-ing thymus cells from a mouse carrying MCA-1490, and they had found that it makes a monoclonal suppressor factor (180,181). The anti-idiotypic MAb 4.72 (which related to sarcoma MCA-1490) was shown to bind to this factor, suggest-ing that anti-idiotypic MAb might be used to counteract the suppressor-cell-mediated inhibition of antitumor reactivity. Furthermore, MAb 4.72 and 5.96 could be used to isolate tumor-reactive lymphocytes from mice bearing the respective tumors. After the lymphocytes had been cultured in vitro, they were found to induce tumor-specific DTH and to have antitumor activity in vivo (176). An analogous approach might be developed to select tumor-reactive lymphocyte populations in human cancer patients, expand them in vitro, and inject them back into the patients. This may have practical advantages over using tumor-infiltrating lymphocytes (39) for cancer therapy.

Lee et al. investigated immunity to mouse bladder carcinomas (178). Rat MAb 6.10 was made which recognizes p175, a glycoprotein expressed strongly on mouse bladder carcinomas and weakly on some normal adult mouse cells. This glycoprotein is also expressed relatively strongly on certain cells from mouse fetuses (182). The p175 antigen is thus analogous to the tumor-associated

antigens most commonly seen in human neoplasms. Two anti-idiotypic MAb relating to p175 were obtained by immunizing mice with MAb 6.10 (178). Both of these anti-idiotypic MAb could induce cell-mediated immunity to syngeneic mouse bladder carcinomas. The cell-mediated immunity was detected in vivo by DTH testing and in vitro by a leukocyte adherence inhibition (LAI) assay (183). The LAI assay measures the reactivity of Lyt-1 positive helper cells and provides a correlate of the DTH reaction (28). No humoral antibodies to p175 were induced. Although antibodies ("Ab3") were present in the sera of mice given either anti-idiotypic MAb and bound to the respective anti-idiotypic MAb, they did not bind to p175 (172). The study by Lee et al. (178) is important because it demonstrates that p175 can induce cell-mediated antitumor immunity in mice, including potentially beneficial DTH reactions, although it is a differentiation ("self") antigen. Consequently, "self" antigens in human neoplasms may induce effective antitumor immunity, if an anti-idiotypic vaccine is used.

Kuchroo et al. (183) further analyzed the immunity of mice to p175 by using the two anti-idiotypic MAb of Lee et al. (178) and performing in vitro tests with the LAI assay. Reactivity to p175 was demonstrated by exposing lymphocytes from mice with bladder carcinomas to antigen extracts containing p175. This reactivity was suppressed by sera from mice with bladder carcinoma but not by sera from mice with a non-cross-reacting tumor, sarcoma MCA-1511. If one of the two bladder carcinoma-related anti-idiotypic MAb was mixed with sera from mice with bladder carcinoma, the ability of the latter sera to suppress LAI reactivity was abolished (183). This is most likely because the anti-idiotypic MAb bound to serum factors responsible for the suppressive effect. By studying, in parallel, mice with either bladder carcinoma or sarcoma MCA-1511, and using anti-idiotypic MAb relating to either p175 or MCA-1511 as an immunoadsorbent, suppressor factors relating to either tumor were specifically isolated. This binding of anti-idiotypic MAb to specific suppressor factors may be utilized toward developing therapeutic protocols aiming to decrease the impact of suppression on the development of effective tumor immunity.

We would like to end this discussion by commenting on two series of experiments which remain relevant although they were done some 15 years ago.

Bansal and Sjögren observed that lymphocytes from rats with growing polyoma tumors were specifically cytolytic to polyoma tumor cells in vitro, and that sera from the rats could specifically suppress ("block") this effect (184). They then hyperimmunized rats against antigens expressed on polyoma tumors and found that the hyperimmune sera abrogated ("unblocked") the "blocking" activity of sera from rats with growing polyoma tumors (184-186), similarly to what had been previously found in a mouse sarcoma system (187). Intravenous injection of the "unblocking" sera induced regression of both primary and transplanted polyoma tumors, including the regression of micro-metastases in

the lung. Some of the treated rats were permanently cured (184–186). As we have discussed in more detail elsewhere (33,174,188), the "unblocking" phenomenon is probably the result of anti-idiotypic antibodies: Analogous "unblocking" sera have been found to contain antibodies to circulating suppressor factors, but not usually to tumor antigens (188,189). Furthermore, the protocol of Bansal and Sjögren to obtain "unblocking" rat antibodies was the one adapted by Nelson's group to obtain the hybridomas shown to make anti-idiotypic MAb (175,176), which, indeed, had "unblocking" characteristics when tested in vitro. We believe that the effects observed by Bansal and Sjögren were mediated by anti-idiotypic antibodies, even if we cannot exclude the possibility that antibodies to tumor antigens were involved.

Horn and Horn reported on a preliminary clinical study on a patient with renal cell carcinoma (190), and continued this work by collaborating with our group (as discussed in Ref. 191). Two of Horn's patients had renal carcinoma metastatic to the lung, and one patient had been cured of renal carcinoma. Lymphocytes from the two patients with progressive disease were cytotoxic to cultured renal carcinoma cells, and sera from these patients suppressed the lymphocyte effect. Serum from the cured patient, on the other hand, was "unblocking," that is, it abrogated the suppressive activity of sera from the two tumor patients. Following infusion of "unblocking" serum from the cured patient to the two tumor-bearing patients, the suppressive activity of sera from these two patients decreased. It is noteworthy that both these patients underwent partial remission of their lung metastases as detected by x-ray examinaion (190,191, L. Horn, personal communication). Although both patients ultimately died of brain metastases, autopsy indicated the disappearance of tumor in several areas originally known to be involved. Because the clinical trial consisted of only two tumor-bearing patients, both of whom ultimately died of their tumors, and whereas renal carcinomas are known to sometimes undergo spontaneous remission, no definitive conclusions can be drawn from this work, but it remains provocative nevertheless. As reviewed a few years ago (192), there are other intriguing but inconclusive reports on patients infused with putative immune sera. These reports include claims that a few patients treated with sera from donors cured of cancer, or with sera from hyperimmunized animals, underwent extensive tumor regression and were cured.

Human trials with anti-idiotypic MAb are likely to be performed over the next several years. They are needed before one can make judgments about the therapeutic efficiency of this approach.

IX. CONCLUSIONS

Human neoplasms express a variety of tumor-associated differentiation antigens, some of which are present at substantially higher levels than in normal cells from the adult host. These antigens may be the targets for therapy by infusion of MAb. A few of the antigens may, in addition, be potential targets for active immunotherapy (therapeutic vaccination).

MAb to tumor-associated antigens may be clinically useful for tumor targeting of therapeutic agents, such as chemotherapeutic drugs, toxins, and radioisotopes, and may have antitumor activity by mediating ADCC and/or CDC. Some clinical benefit has been observed in patients treated with unmodified mouse MAb, and there is evidence suggesting that a host response is induced to antigens and is responsible for this benefit. Chimeric (mouse–human) antibodies, and MAb which are entirely human, are likely to be less immunogenic in humans and should lend themselves better than mouse MAb to repeated use in the same patient. They are also effective mediators of ADCC and CDC, even at concentrations which should be achievable throughout tumor tissue following intravenous administration of the antibody.

That patients can form immune responses to some tumor-associated differentiation antigens implies that the organism is not tolerant to all of these antigens, even though the antigens are present at trace levels on normal cells. Some encouraging observations toward tumor immunization have been made in animal models using either live recombinant viruses or treatment with anti-idiotypic MAb. However, elimination of substantial tumor masses appears to be difficult to achieve. Procedures which counteract the down-regulatory roles of suppressor cells and their factors might be useful in this context. One may, for example, strive for selective inhibition of tumor-antigen-specific suppression, and for obtaining populations of tumor-antigen-specific lymphocytes which have reached a state of activation where they can no longer be suppressed. Anti-idiotypic MAb may be helpful for this purpose. A potentially useful model system for developing various approaches toward active immunotherapy is provided by mouse tumor lines which express the human p97 antigen following transfection. One then has available large amounts of soluble tumor antigen, many antitumor MAb of different isotypes, a recombinant live virus vaccine, and several anti-idiotypic MAb.

We conclude that treatment with antitumor MAb, biologically functional themselves, and given alone or together with immunomodulators, as well as treatment with radiolabeled MAb and conjugates between MAb and chemotherapeutic drugs, is likely to become clinically useful, although there is still a far way to go. We also conclude that active immunization with recombinant vaccines and/or anti-idiotypic MAb has potential for the elimination of those tumor cells which may remain after primary cancer therapy.

ACKNOWLEDGMENTS

The authors wish to acknowledge collaboration with Drs. P. L. Beaumier, J. P. Brown, C. D. Estin, G. E. Goodman, S. M. Larson, V. L. Lee, A. Y. Liu, K. A. Nelson, G. T. Nepom, G. D. Plowman, R. R. Robinson, and M. Y. Yeh. Our thanks are also due to Mrs. Phyllis Harps for preparing the manuscript, and Drs. H. P. Fell, J. A. Ledbetter, P. S. Linsley, and P. D. Senter for reading it critically. The recent work by the authors has been supported by ONCOGEN, and (with respect to human melanoma) by National Institutes of Health Grant CA 38011.

REFERENCES

1. Klein, G. and Klein, E. (1977). Rejectability of virus-induced tumors and nonrejectability of spontaneous tumors. *Transplant. Proc. 9*: 1095–1104.
2. Abelev, G. I., Perova, S. D., Khramkova, N. I., Postinihova, Z. A., Irlin, I. S. (1963). Production of embryonal beta-globulin by transplantable mouse hepatomas. *Transplantation 1*: 174–180.
3. Gold, P., and Freedman, S. O. (1965). Specific carcinoembryonic antigens of the human digestive system. *J. Exp. Med. 122*: 467–481.
4. Hellström, K. E., Hellström, I., and Goodman, G. E. (1987). Antibodies for drug delivery. In: *Controlled Drug Delivery, Fundamentals and Applications*. Edited by J. R. Robinson and V. H. L. Lee. Marcel Dekker, New York and Basel, pp. 623–653.
5. Hellström, I., Hellström, K. E., Pierce, G. E., and Yang, J. P. S. (1968). Cellular and humoral immunity to different types of human neoplasms. *Nature 220*: 1352–1354.
6. Hellström, I., Hellström, K. E., Sjögren, H. O., and Warner, G. A. (1971). Demonstration of cell-mediated immunity to human neoplasms of various histological types. *Int. J. Cancer 7*: 1–16.
7. Bubenik, J., Perlman, P., Helmstein, K., and Moberger, G. (1970). Cellular and humoral immune responses to human urinary bladder carcinomas. *Int. J. Cancer 5*: 310–319.
8. Hellström, K. E., and Hellström, I. (1969). Cellular immunity against tumor specific antigens. *Adv. Cancer Res. 12*: 167–223.
9. Hellström, I., and Hellström, K. E. (1973). Some recent studies on cellular immunity to human melanomas. *Fed. Proc. 32*: 156–159.
10. Hellström, I., Hellström, K. E., and Shepard, T. H. (1970). Cell-mediated immunity against antigens common to human colonic carcinomas and fetal gut epithelium. *Int. J. Cancer 6*: 346–351.
11. Lewis, M. G., Ikonopisov, R. L., Nairn, R. C., Phillips, T. M., Hamilton-Fairly, G., Bodenham, D. C., and Alexander, P. (1969). Tumor-specific antibodies in human malignant melanoma and their relationship to extent of disease. *Br. Med. J. 3*: 547–552.

12. Morton, D. L., Malmgren, R. A., Holmes, E. C., and Ketcham, A. S. (1968). Demonstration of antibodies against human malignant melanoma by immunofluorescence. *Surgery, St. Louis 64*: 233–240.
13. Cornain, S., deVries, J. E., Collard, J., Vennegoor, C., Wingerden, I. V., and Rumke, P. (1975). Antibodies and antigen expression in human melanoma detected by the immune adherence test. *Int. J. Cancer 16*: 981–997.
14. Shiku, H., Takahashi, T., Oettgen, H. F., and Old, L. J. (1976). Cell surface antigens of human malignant melanoma: II. Serological typing with immune adherence assays and definition of two new surface antigens. *J. Exp. Med. 144*: 873–881.
15. Real, F. X., Mattes, M. J., Houghton, A. N., Oettgen, H. F., Lloyd, K. O., and Old, L. J. (1984). Class 1 (unique) tumor antigens of human melanoma. Identification of a 90,000 dalton cell surface glycoprotein by autologous antibody. *J. Exp. Med. 160*: 1219–1233.
16. Vanky, F., Klein, E., Willems, J., Book, K., Ivert, T., Peterffy, A., Nilsonne, U., and Kreicbergs, A. (1987). Lysis of autologous tumor cells by blood lymphocytes activated in autologous mixed lymphocyte tumor cell culture—no correlation with the postsurgical clinical course. *Cancer Immunol. Immunother. 24*: 180–183.
17. Mukherji, B., Guha, A., Loomis, R., and Ergin, M. T. (1987). Cell-mediated amplification and down regulation of cytotoxic immune response against autologous human cancer. *J. Immunol. 138*: 1987–1991.
18. Herberman, R. B., and Oldham, R. K. (1975). Problems associated with study of cell-mediated immunity to human tumor by microcytotoxicity assays. *J. Natl. Cancer Inst. 55*: 749–753.
19. Cannon, G. B., Bonnard, G. D., Djeu, J., West, W. H., and Herberman, R. B. (1977). Relationship of human natural lymphocyte-mediated cytotoxicity to cytotoxicity of breast-cancer-derived target cells. *Int. J. Cancer 19*: 487–497.
20. Steele, G., Sjögren, H. O., and Stadenberg, I. (1976). In vitro cell-mediated immune reactions of melanoma in colorectal carcinoma patients demonstrated by long-term chromium assays. *Int. J. Cancer 17*: 27–39.
21. DeVries, J. E., and Spitz, H. (1984). Cloned human cytotoxic T lymphocyte (CTL) lines reactive with autologous melanoma cells. In vitro generation, isolation, and analysis to phenotype and specificity. *J. Immunol. 132*: 510–519.
22. Hellström, I., and Hellström, K. E. (1983). Cell-mediated reactivity to human tumor-type associated antigens: Does it Exist? *J. Biol. Resp. Modifiers 2*: 310–320.
23. Taranger, L. A., Chapman, W. H., Hellström, I., and Hellström, K. E. (1972). Immunological studies on urinary bladder tumors of rats and mice. *Science 176*: 1337–1340.
24. Steele, G., Jr., Sjögren, H. O., Rosengren, J. E., Linstrom, C., Larsson, A., and Leandoer, L. (1975). Sequential studies of serum blocking activity in rats bearing chemically induced primary bowel tumors. *J. Natl. Cancer Inst. 54*: 959–967.

25. McCoy, J. L., Jerome, L. F., Dean, J. H., Cannon, G. B., Alford, T. C., Doering, T., and Herberman, R. B. (1974). Inhibition of leukocyte migration by tumor-associated antigens in soluble extracts of human breast carcinoma. *J. Natl. Cancer Inst. 53*: 11-17.
26. McCoy, J. L., Jerome, L. F., Dean, J. H., Perlin, E., Oldham, R. K., Char, D. H., Cohen, M. H., Felix, E. L., and Herberman, R. B. (1975). Inhibition of leukocyte migration by tumor-associated antigens in soluble extracts of human malignant melanoma. *J. Natl. Cancer Inst. 55*: 19-24.
27. McCoy, J. L., Jerome, L. F., Cannon, G. B., Weese, J. L., and Herberman, R. B. (1977). Reactivity of lung cancer patients in leukocyte migration inhibition assays to 3-M potassium chloride extracts of fresh tumor and tissue-cultured cells derived from lung cancer. *J. Natl. Cancer Inst. 59*: 1413-1418.
28. International Workshop on Leukocyte Adherence Inhibition, Roswell Park Memorial Institute. (1979). *Cancer Res. 39*: 551-662.
29. Kall, M. A., Hellström, I., and Hellström, K. E. (1975). Different responses of lymphoid cells from tumor-bearing as compared to tumor-immunized mice when sensitized to tumor specific antigens in vitro. *Proc. Natl. Acad. Sci. USA 72*: 5086-5089.
30. Greene, M. I., Martin, E. D., Pierres, M., and Benacerraf, B. (1977). Reduction of syngeneic tumor growth by an anti-IJ-alloantiserum. *Proc. Natl. Acad. Sci. USA 75*: 5118-5121.
31. Hellström, K. E., Hellström, I., Kant, J. A., and Tamerius, J. D. (1978). Regression and inhibition of sarcoma growth by interference with a radiosensitive T cell population. *J. Exp. Med. 148*: 799-804.
32. North, R. J. (1986). Radiation induced, immunologically mediated regression of an established tumor as an example of successful therapeutic immunomanipulation. Preferential elimination of suppressor T cells allows sustained production of effector T cells. *J. Exp. Med. 164*: 1652-1666.
33. Nepom, G. T., Hellström, I., and Hellström, K. E. (1983). Suppressor mechanisms in tumor immunity. *Experientia 39*: 235-242.
34. Hellström, I., Hellström, K. E., Evans, C. A., Heppner, G., Pierce, G. E., and Yang, J. P. S. (1969). Serum mediated protection of neoplastic cells from inhibition by lymphocytes immune to their tumor specific antigens. *Proc. Natl. Acad. Sci. USA 62*: 362-369.
35. Hellström, I., Hellström, K. E., and Nelson, K. (1983). Antigen-specific suppressor ("blocking") factors in tumor immunity. In: *Biomembranes*. Edited by A. Nowotny. Plenum Press, New York, Vol. 11, pp. 365-388.
36. Hellström, K. E., Hellström, I., Snyder, H. W., Jr., Balin, J. P., and Jones, F. R. (1985). Blocking ("suppressor") factors, immune complexes and extracorporeal immunoadsorption in tumor immunity. In *Immune Complexes and Cancer*. Edited by F. A. Salinas and M. G. Hanna, Jr. Plenum Press, New York, pp. 213-238.
37. Hellström, K. E., and Hellström, I. (1974). Lymphocyte-mediated cytotoxicity and blocking serum activity to tumor antigens. In *Advances in Immunology*, Vol. 18. Edited by F. J. Dixon, Academic Press, Inc., New York, pp. 209-277.

38. Rosenberg, S. A., Lotze, M. T., Muul, L. M., Leitman, S., Chang, A. E., Ettinghausen, S. E., Matory, Y. L., Skibber, J. M., Shiloni, E., Vetto, J. T., et al. (1985). Observations on the systemic administration of autologous lymphokine-activated killer cells and recombinant interleukin-2 to patients with metastatic cancer. *N. Engl. J. Med. 313*: 1485–1492.

39. Rosenberg, S. A., Spiess, P., and Lafreniere, R. (1986). A new approach to the adoptive immunotherapy of cancer with tumor-infiltrating lymphocytes. *Science 233*: 1318–1321.

40. Kohler, G., and Milstein, C. (1975). Continuous culture of fused cells secreting antibodies of predefined specificity. *Nature 256*: 495–497.

41. Sears, H. F., Mattis, J., Herlyn, D., Hayry, P., Atkinson, B., Ernst, C., Steplewski, Z., and Koprowski, H. (1982). Phase I clinical trial of monoclonal antibody in treatment of gastrointestinal tumors. *Lancet 1*: 762–765.

42. Houghton, A. N., Mintzer, D., Cordon-Cardo, C., Welt, S., Fliegel, B., Vadham, S., Carswell, E., Melamed, M. R., Otettgen, H. F., and Old, L. J. (1985). Mouse monoclonal IgG3 antibody detecting GD3 ganglioside—A Phase I trial in patients with malignant melanoma. *Proc. Natl. Acad. Sci. USA 82*: 1242–1246.

43. Sears, H. F., Herlyn, D., Steplewski, Z., and Koprowski, H. (1986). Initial trial use of murine monoclonal antibodies as immunotherapeutic agents for gastrointestinal adenocarcinoma. *Hybridoma 5* (Suppl. 1): S109–115.

44. Koprowski, H., Herlyn, D., Lubeck, M., DeFreitas, E., and Sears, H. F. (1984). Human anti-idiotype antibodies in cancer patients: Is the modulation of the immune response beneficial for the patient. *Proc. Natl. Acad. Sci. USA 81*: 216–219.

45. Woodbury, R. G., Brown, J. P., Yeh, M-Y., Hellström, I., and Hellström, K. E. (1980). Identification of a cell surface protein, p97, in human melanomas and certain other neoplasms. *Proc. Natl. Acad. Sci. USA 77*: 2183–2186.

46. Dippold, W. G., Lloyd, K. O., Li, L. T. C., Ikeda, H., Oettgen, H. F., and Old, L. J. (1980). Cell surface antigens of human malignant melanoma: Definition of six antigenic systems with mouse monoclonal antibodies. *Proc. Natl. Acad. Sci. USA 77*: 6114–6118.

47. Brown, J. P., Nishiyama, K., Hellström, I., and Hellström, K. E. (1981). Structural characterization of human melanoma-associated antigen p97 using monoclonal antibodies. *J. Immunol. 127*: 539–546.

48. Khosravi, M. J., Dent, P. B., and Liao, S.-K. (1985). Structural characterization and biosynthesis of gp87, a melanoma-associated oncofetal antigen defined by monoclonal antibody. *Int. J. Cancer 35*: 73–80.

49. Brown, J. P., Wright, P. W., Hart, C. E., Woodbury, R. G., Hellström, K. E., and Hellström, I. (1980). Protein antigens of normal and malignant tumor cells identified by immunoprecipitation with monoclonal antibodies. *J. Biol. Chem. 255*: 4980–4983.

50. Brown, J. P., Woodbury, R. G., Hart, C. E., Hellström, I., and Hellström, K. E. (1981). Quantitative analysis of melanoma-associated antigen p97 in normal and neoplastic tissues. *Proc. Natl. Acad. Sci. USA 78*: 539–543.

51. Woodbury, R. G., Brown, J. P., Loop, S. M., Hellström, K. E., and Hellström, I. (1981). Analysis of normal and neoplastic human tissues for the tumor-associated protein p97. *Int. J. Cancer 27*: 145–149.

52. Bageshaw, K. D. (1983). Tumour markers—where do we go from here? Third Gordon Hamilton-Fairley Memorial Lecture. *Br. J. Cancer 48*: 167–175.

53. Hellström, K. E., and Hellström, I. (1985). Monoclonal anti-melanoma antibodies and their possible clinical use. In *Monoclonal Antibodies for Tumour Detection and Drug Targeting*. Edited by R. W. Baldwin and V. S. Byers. Academic Press, New York, pp. 17–51.

54. Brown, J. P., Hewick, R. M., Hellström, I., Hellström, K. E., Doolittle, R. F., and Dreyer, W. J. (1982). Human melanoma-associated antigen p97 is structurally and functionally related to transferrin. *Nature 296*: 171–173.

55. Plowman, G. D., Brown, J. P., Enns, C. A., Schröder, J., Nikinmaa, B., Sussman, H. H., Hellström, K. E., and Hellström, I. (1983). Assignment of the gene for human melanoma-associated antigen p97 to chromosome 3. *Nature 303*: 70–72.

56. Yang, F., Lum, J. B., McGill, J. R., Moore, C. M., Naylor, S. L., van Bragt, P. H., Baldwin, W. D., and Bowman, B. H. (1984). Human transferrin: cDNA characterization and chromosomal localization. *Proc. Natl. Acad. Sci. USA 81*: 2752–2756.

57. Brown, J. P., Rose, T. M., Forstrom, J. W., Hellström, I., and Hellström, K. E. (1985). Isolation of cDNA clone for human melanoma-associated antigen p97. In *Molecular Biology of Tumor Cells*. Edited by B. Wahren. Raven Press, New York, pp. 157–167.

58. Rose, T. M., Plowman, G. D., Teplow, D. B., Dreyer, W. J., Hellström, K. E., and Brown, J. P. (1986). Primary structure of the human melanoma-associated antigen p97 (melanotransferrin) deduced from the mRNA sequence. *Proc. Natl. Acad. Sci. USA 83*: 1261–1265.

59. Plowman, G. D. (1986). Characterization and expression of the melanotransferrin (p97) gene. Ph.D. dissertation, University of Washington.

60. Estin, C. D., Stevenson, U., Kahn, M., Hellström, I., and Hellström, K. E. Transfected mouse melanoma lines expressing varying levels of human melanoma-associated p97. Submitted for publication.

61. Fidler, I. J., and Hart, I. R. (1981). Biological and experimental consequences of the zonal composition of solid tumors. *Cancer Res. 41*: 3266–3267.

62. Beaumier, P., Krohn, K., Carrasquillo, J., Eary, J., Hellström, K. E., Hellström, I., Nelp, W., and Larson, W. (1985). Melanoma localization in nude mice with monoclonal Fab against p97. *J. Nucl. Med. 26*: 1172–1179.

63. Larson, S. M., Brown, J. P., Wright, P. W., Carrasquillo, J. A., Hellström, I., and Hellström, K. E. (1983). Imaging of melanoma with ^{131}I-labeled monoclonal antibodies. *J. Nucl. Med. 24*: 123–129.

64. Larson, S. M., Carrasquillo, J. A., Krohn, K. A., McGuffin, R. W., Hellström, I., Hellström, K. E., and Lyster, D. (1983). Diagnostic imaging of malignant melanoma with radiolabeled anti-tumor antibodies. *J. Am. Med. Assoc. 249*: 811–812.

65. Larson, S. M., Carrasquillo, J. A., Krohn, K. A., Brown, J. P., McGuffin, R. W., Ferens, J. M., Graham, M. M., Hill, L. D., Beaumier, P. L., Hellström, K. E., and Hellström, I. (1983). Localization of p97 specific Fab fragments in human melanoma as a basis for radiotherapy. *J. Clin. Invest. 72*: 2101–2114.

66. Carrasquillo, J. A., Krohn, K. A., Beaumier, P., McGuffin, R. W., Brown, J. P., Hellström, K. E., Hellström, I., and Larson, S. M. (1984). Diagnosis and therapy of solid tumors with radiolabelled Fab. *Cancer Treat. Rep. 68*: 317–328.

67. Delaloye, B., Bischof-Delaloye, A., Buchegger, F., von Fliedner, V., Grob, J. P., Volant, J. C., Pettavel, J., and Mach, J. P. (1986). Detection of colorectal carcinoma by emission-computerized tomography after injection of ^{123}I-labeled Fab or F(ab')$_2$ fragments from monoclonal anti-carcinoembryonic antigen antibodies. *J. Clin. Invest. 77*: 301–311.

68. Siccardi, A. G., Buraggi, G. L., Callegaro, L., Mariani, G., Natali, P. G., Abbati, A., Bestagno, M., Caputo, V., Mansi, L., Masi, R., Paganelli, G., Riva, P., Salvatore, M., Sanguineti, M., Troncone, L., Turco, G. L., Scassellati, G. A., and Ferrone, S. (1986). Multicenter study of immunoscintigraphy with radiolabelled monoclonal antibodies in patients with melanoma. *Cancer Res. 46*: 4817–4822.

69. Goodman, G. E., Beaumier, P. L., Hellström, I., Fernyhough, B., and Hellström, K. E. (1985). Pilot trial of murine monoclonal antibodies in patients with advanced melanoma. *J. Clin. Oncol. 3*: 340–352.

70. Hellström, I., Brankovan, V., and Hellström, K. E. (1985). Strong antitumor activities of IgG3 antibodies to a human melanoma-associated ganglioside. *Proc. Natl. Acad. Sci. USA 82*: 1499–1502.

71. Hellström, I., Garrigues, H. J., Cabasco, L., Mosely, G. H., Brown, J. P., and Hellström, K. E. (1983). Studies of a high molecular weight human melanoma-associated antigen. *J. Immunol. 130*: 1467–1472.

72. Hellström, I., Brown, J. P., and Hellström, K. E. (1981). Monoclonal antibodies to two determinants of melanoma-antigen p97 act synergistically in complement-dependent cytotoxicity. *J. Immunol. 127*: 157–160.

73. Casellas, P., Brown, J. P., Gros, O., Gros, P., Hellström, I., Jansen, F. K., Poncelet, P., Vidal, H., and Hellström, K. E. (1982). Human melanoma cells can be killed in vitro by an immunotoxin specific for melanoma-associated antigen p97. *Int. J. Cancer 30*: 437–443.

74. Rowland, G. F., Axton, C. A., Baldwin, R. W., Brown, J. P., Corvalan, J. R. F., Embleton, M. J., Gore, V. A., Hellström, I., Hellström, K. E., Jacobs, E., Marsden, C. H., Pimm, M. V., Simmonds, R. G., and Smith, W. (1985). Anti-tumor properties of vindesine-monoclonal antibody conjugates. *Cancer Immunol. Immunother. 19*: 1–7.

75. Nepom, G. T., Nelson, K. A., Holbeck, S. L., Hellström, I., and Hellström, K. E. (1984). Induction of immunity to a human tumor marker by in vivo administration of anti-idiotypic antibodies in mice. *Proc. Natl. Acad. Sci. USA 81*: 2864–2867.

76. Estin, C. D., Stevenson, U. S., Plowman, G. D., Ju, S.-L., Sridhar, P., Hellström, I., Hellström, K. E., and Brown, J. P. (1988). Recombinant vaccinia vaccine against the human melanoma antigen p97 for use in immunotherapy. *Proc. Natl. Acad. Sci. USA 85*: 1052–1056.

77. Gown, A. M., and Vogel, A. M. (1985). Monoclonal antibodies to human intermediate filament proteins. III. Analysis of tumors. *Am. J. Clin. Pathol. 84*: 413–424.

78. Welt, S., Mattes, M. J., Grando, R., Thomson, T. M., Leonard, R. W., Zanzonico, P. B., Bigler, R. E., Yeh, S., Oettgen, H. F., and Old, L. J. (1987). Monoclonal antibody to an intracellular antigen images human melanoma transplants in nu/nu mice. *Proc. Natl. Acad. Sci. USA 84*: 1200–4204.

79. East, I. J., Keenan, A. M., Larson, S. M., and Dean, J. (1984). Scintigraphy of normal mouse ovaries with monoclonal antibodies to ZP-2, the major zona pellucida protein. *Science 225*: 938–941.

80. Meeker, T., Lowder, J., Cleary, M. L., Stewart, S., Warnke, R., Sklar, J., and Levy, R. (1985). Emergence of idiotype variants during treatment of B cell lymphoma with anti-idiotype antibodies. *N. Engl. J. Med. 312*: 1658–1665.

81. Lowder, J. N., Meeker, T. C., and Levy, R. (1985). Monoclonal antibody therapy of lymphoid malignancy. *Cancer Surv. 1*: 359–375.

82. Miller, R. A., Lowder, J., Meeker, T. C., Brown, S., Levy, R. (1987). Anti-idiotypes in B-cell tumor therapy. *NCI Monogr. 3*: 131–134.

83. Lowder, J. M., Meeker, T. C., Campbell, M., Carcia, C. F., Gralow, J., Miller, R. A., Warnke, R., and Levy, R. (1987). Studies on B lymphoid tumors treated with monoclonal anti-idiotype antibodies: correlation with clinical responses. *Blood 69*: 199–210.

84. Carroll, W. L., Lowder, J. N., Streifer, R., Warnke, R., Levy, S., and Levy, R. (1986). Idiotype variant cell populations in patients with B cell lymphoma. *J. Exp. Med. 164*: 1566–1580.

85. Bumol, T. F., and Reisfeld, R. A. (1982). Unique glycoprotein–proteoglycan complex defined by monoclonal antibody on human melanoma cells. *Proc. Natl. Acad. Sci. USA 79*: 1245–1249.

86. Koprowski, H., and Steplewski, Z. (1981). Human solid tumor antigens defined by monoclonal antibodies. In *Monoclonal Antibodies and T-Cell Hybridomas*. Edited by G. J. Hammerling, U. Hammerling, and J. F. Kearney. Elsevier/North-Holland Biomedical Press, Amsterdam, pp. 161–173.

87. Rakowicz-Szulczynska, E. M., Rodeck, U., Herlyn, M., and Koprowski, H. (1986). Chromatin binding of epidermal growth factor, nerve growth factors, and platelet-derived growth factor in cells bearing the appropriate surface receptors. *Proc. Natl. Acad. Sci. USA 83*: 3728–3732.

32 Hellström and Hellström

88. Loop, S. M., Nishiyama, K., Hellström, I., Woodbury, R. G., Brown, J. P., and Hellström, K. E. (1981). Two human tumor-associated antigens, p155 and p210, detected by monoclonal antibodies. *Int. J. Cancer 27*: 775–781.
89. Yeh, M.-Y., Hellström, I., Abe, K., Hakomori, S., and Hellström, K. E. (1982). A cell surface antigen which is present in the ganglioside fraction and shared by human melanomas. *Int. J. Cancer 29*: 269–275.
90. Tsuchida, T., Saxton, R. E., Morton, D. L., and Irie, R. F. (1987). Gangliosides of human melanoma. *J. Natl. Cancer Inst. 78*: 45–54.
91. Colcher, D., Horan Hand, P., Nuti, M., and Schlom, J. (1981). A spectrum of monoclonal antibodies reactive with human mammary tumor cells. *Proc. Natl. Acad. Sci. USA 78*: 3199–3203.
92. Cuttitta, F., Rosen, S., Gazdar, A. F., and Minna, J. D. (1981). Monoclonal antibodies that demonstrate specificity for several types of human lung cancer. *Proc. Natl. Acad. Sci. USA 78*: 4591–4595.
93. Varki, N. M., Reisfeld, R. A., and Walker, L. E. (1984). Antigens associated with a human lung adenocarcinoma defined by monoclonal antibodies. *Cancer Res. 44*: 681–687.
94. Fernsten, P. D., Pekny, K. W., Reisfeld, R. A., and Walker, L. E. (1986). Antigens associated with human squamous cell lung carcinoma defined by murine monoclonal antibodies. *Cancer Res. 46*: 2970–2977.
95. Hellström, I., Horn, D., Linsley, P., Brown, J. P., Brankovan, V., and Hellström, K. E. (1986). Monoclonal mouse antibodies raised against human lung carcinoma. *Cancer Res. 46*: 3917–3923.
96. Finstad, C. L., Cordon-Cardo, C., Bander, N. H., Whitmore, W. F., Malamed, M. R., and Old, L. J. (1985). Specificity analysis of mouse monoclonal antibodies defining cell surface antigens of human renal cancer. *Proc. Natl. Acad. Sci. USA 82*: 2955–2959.
97. Embleton, M. J., Gunn, B., Byers, V. S., and Baldwin, R. W. (1981). Antitumour reactions of monoclonal antibody against a human osteogenic-sarcoma cell line. *Br. J. Cancer 43*: 582–587.
98. Ritz, J., Pesando, J. M., Notis-McConarty, J., Clavell, L. A., Sallan, S. E., and Schlossman, S. F. (1981). Use of monoclonal antibodies as diagnostic and therapeutic reagents in acute lymphoblastic leukemia. *Cancer Res. 41*: 4771.
99. Clark, E. A., Shu, G., and Ledbetter, J. A. (1985). Role of Bp35 cell surface polypeptide in human B-cell activation. *Proc. Natl. Acad. Sci. USA 82*: 1766–1770.
100. Ledbetter, J. A., Shu, G., Gallagher, M., and Clark, E. A. (1987). Augmentation of normal and malignant B cell proliferation by monoclonal antibody to the B cell-specific antigen Bp50 (CDW40). *J. Immunol. 138*: 788–794.
101. Wright, G. L., Jr. (Ed.) (1984). *Monoclonal Antibodies and Cancer, Immunology Series 23*. Marcel Dekker, Inc., New York.
102. Reisfeld, R. A., and Sell, S. (Eds.) (1985). *Monoclonal Antibodies and Cancer Therapy*, UCLA Symposia on Molecular and Cellular Biology, New Series, Vol. 27. Alan R. Liss, Inc., New York.

103. Baldwin, R. W., and Byers, V. S. (Eds.) (1985). *Monoclonal Antibodies for Tumour Detection and Drug Targeting*. Academic Press, New York, pp. 17–51.
104. Roth, J. A. (Ed.) (1986). *Monoclonal Antibodies for the Diagnosis and Therapy of Cancer*. Futura Publishing, Mt. Kisco, New York.
105. Reisfeld, R. A. (1986). Immunochemical characterization of human tumor antigen. *Semin. Oncol. 13*: 153–164.
106. Vollmers, H. P., and Birchmeier, W. (1983). Monoclonal antibodies inhibit the adhesion of mouse B16 melanoma cells in vitro and block lung metastases in vivo. *Proc. Natl. Acad. Sci. USA 80*: 3729–3733.
107. Vollmers, H. P., and Birchmeier, W. (1983). Monoclonal antibodies that prevent adhesion of B16 melanoma cells and reduce metastases in mice: Crossreaction with human tumor cells. *Proc. Natl. Acad. Sci. USA 80*: 6863–6867.
108. Hellström, I., Beaumier, P. L., and Hellström, K. E. (1986). Antitumor effects of L6, and IgG2a antibody reacting with most human carcinomas. *Proc. Natl. Acad. Sci. USA 83*: 7059–7063.
109. Schultz, G., Staffileno, L. K., Reisfeld, R. A., and Dennert, G. (1985). Eradication of established human melanoma tumors in nude mice by antibody-directed effector cells. *J. Exp. Med. 161*: 1315–1325.
110. Herberman, R. B., Morgan, A. C., Reisfeld, R. A., Cheresh, D. A., and Ortaldo, J. R. (1985). Antibody-dependent cellular cytotoxicity (ADCC) against human melanoma by human effector cells in cooperation with mouse monoclonal antibodies. In *Monoclonal Antibodies and Cancer Therapy*. UCLA Symposia on Molecular and Cellular Biology, New Series, Vol. 27. Edited by R. A. Reisfeld and S. Sell. Alan R. Liss, Inc., New York, pp. 193–203.
111. Johnson, W. J., Steplewski, Z., Matthews, T. J., Hamilton, T. A., Koprowski, H., and Adams, D. O. (1986). Cytolytic interactions between macrophages, tumor cells, and monoclonal antibodies: Characterization of lytic conditions and requirements for effector activation. *J. Immunol. 136*: 4704–4713.
112. Hellström, I., Garrigues, U., Lavie, E., and Hellström, K. E. (1988). Antibody-mediated killing of human tumor cells by attached effector cells. *Cancer Res. 48*: 624–627.
113. Bernstein, I. D., Tam, M. R., and Nowinski, R. C. (1980). Mouse leukemia therapy with monoclonal antibodies against a thymus differentiation antigen. *Science 207*: 68–71.
114. Bernstein, I. D., Nowinski, R. C., Tam, M. R., McMaster, B., Houston, L. L., and Clark, E. A. (1980). Monoclonal antibody therapy of mouse leukemia. In *Monoclonal Antibodies*. Edited by R. H. Kennett, T. C. McKearn, and K. B. Pechtol. Plenum Press, New York, pp. 275–291.
115. Goodman, G. E., Yen, Y.-P., Cox, T. C., Hellström, K. E., and Hellström, I. (1987). The effect of monoclonal antibody MG-21 plus human complement on in vitro cloning of fresh human melanoma. *Proc. of the 78th Ann. Meet. Am. Assoc. Cancer Res. 28*, 389.

116. Hellström, K. E., Hellström, I., Goodman, G. E., and Brankovan, V. (1985). Antibody-dependent cellular cytotoxicity to human melanoma antigens. In *Monoclonal Antibodies and Cancer Therapy*. UCLA Symposia on Molecular and Cellular Biology, New Series. Edited by R. A. Reisfeld and S. Sell. Alan R. Liss, Inc., New York, pp. 149–164.

117. Honsik, C. J., Jung, G., and Reisfeld, R. A. (1986). Lymphokine-activated killer cells targeted by monoclonal antibodies to the disialogangliosides GD2 and GD3 specifically lyse human tumor cells of neuroectodermal origin. *Proc. Natl. Acad. Sci. USA 83*: 7893–7897.

118. Irie, R. F., and Morton, D. L. (1986). Regression of cutaneous metastatic melanoma by intralesional injection with human monoclonal antibody to ganglioside GD2. *Proc. Natl. Acad. Sci. USA 83*: 8695–8698.

119. Sindelar, W. F., Maher, M. M., Herlyn, D., Sears, H. F., Steplewski, H., and Koprowski, H. (1986). Trial of therapy with monoclonal antibody 17-1A in pancreatic carcinoma: preliminary results. *Hybridoma 5* (Suppl. 1). S125–132.

120. Steplewski, Z., Sears, H. F., and Koprowski, H. (1986). Monoclonal antibody infusion in gastrointestinal cancer patients. *Rec. Res. Cancer Res. 100*: 321–333.

121. Knuth, A., Danowski, B., Oettgen, H. F., and Old, L. J. (1984). T cell-mediated cytotoxicity against autologous malignant melanoma: analysis with interleukin 2-dependent T-cell cultures. *Proc. Natl. Acad. Sci. USA 81*: 3511–3515.

122. Lotze, M. T., Carrasquillo, J. A., Weinstein, J. N., Bryant, G. J., Perentesis, P., Reynolds, J. C., Matis, L. A., Eger, R. R., Keenan, A. M., Hellström, I., and Hellström, K. E. (1986). Monoclonal imaging of human melanoma. Radioimmunodetection by subcutaneous or systemic injection. *Ann. Surg. 204*: 223–235.

123. Novotny, J., Handschumacher, M., and Haber, E. (1986). Location of antigenic epitopes on antibody molecules. *J. Mol. Biol. 189*: 715–721.

124. Spira, G., Bargellesi, A., Teillaud, J. L., and Scharff, M. D. (1984). The identification of monoclonal class switch variants by sib-selection and ELISA assay. *J. Immunol. Meth. 74*: 307–315.

125. Cole, S. P. C., Kozbor, D., and Roder, J. C. (1985). The EBV-hybridoma technique and its application to human lung cancer. In *Monoclonal Antibodies and Cancer Therapy*. UCLA Symposia on Molecular and Cellular Biology, New Series, Vol. 27. Edited by R. A. Reisfeld and S. Sell. Alan R. Liss, Inc., New York, pp. 77–96.

126. Glassy, M. C., Gaffar, S. A., Peters, R. E., and Royston, I. (1985). Human monoclonal antibodies to human cancer cells. In *Monoclonal Antibodies and Cancer Therapy*. UCLA Symposia on Molecular and Cellular Biology, New Series, Vol. 27. Edited by R. A. Reisfeld and S. Sell. Alan R. Liss, Inc., New York, pp. 97–109.

127. Cote, R. J., Morrissey, D. M., Houghton, A. N., Beattie, E. J., Jr., Oettgen, H. F., and Old, L. J. (1983). *Proc. Natl. Acad. Sci. USA 80*: 2026–2030.

128. Hellström, K. E., and Brown, J. P. (1979). Tumor antigens. In *The Antigens*, Vol. 5. Edited by M. Sela. Academic Press, New York, pp. 1–82.

129. Morrison, S. L. (1985). Transfectomas provide novel chimeric antibodies. *Science 229*: 1202–1207.

130. Neuberger, M. S., Williams, G. T., and Fox, R. O. (1984). Recombinant antibodies possessing novel effector functions. *Nature 312*: 604–608.

131. Sahagan, B. G., Dorai, H., Saltzgaber-Muller, J., Toneguzzo, F., Guindon, C. A., Lilly, S. P., McDonald, K. W., Morrissey, D. V., Stone, B. A., Davis, G. L., McIntosh, P. K., and Moore, G. P. (1987). A genetically engineered murine/human chimeric antibody retains specificity for human tumor-associated antigen. *J. Immunol. 137*: 1066–1074.

132. Nishimura, Y., Yokoyama, M., Araki, K., Ueda, R., Judo, A., and Watanabe, T. (1987). Recombinant human-mouse chimeric monoclonal antibody specific for common acute lymphocytic leukemia antigen. *Cancer Res. 47*: 999–1005.

133. Sun, L. K., Curtis, P., Rakowicz-Szulczynska, E., Ghrayeb, J., Chang, N., Morrison, S. L., and Koprowski, H. (1987). Chimeric antibody with human constant regions and mouse variable regions directed against carcinoma-associated antigen 17-1A. *Proc. Natl. Acad. Sci. USA 84*: 214–218.

134. Liu, A. Y., Robinson, R. R., Hellström, K. E., Murray, D., Jr., Chang, C. P., and Hellström, I. (1987). Chimeric mouse-human IgG1 antibody that can mediate lysis of cancer cells. *Proc. Natl. Acad. Sci. USA 84*: 3439–3443.

135. Lui, A. Y., Robinson, R. R., Murray, E. D., Jr., Ledbetter, J. A., Hellström, I., and Hellström, K. E. (1987). Production of a mouse-human chimeric MAb to CD20 with potent biological activity. *J. Immunol. 139*: 3521–3526.

136. Ho, D. H., Brown, N. S., Yen, A., Holmes, R., Keating, M., Abuchowski, A., Newman, R. A., and Krakoff, I. H. (1886). Clinical pharmacology of polyethylene glycol-L-asparaginase. *Drug. Metabol. Dispos. 14*: 349–352.

137. De Nardo, S., DeNardo, G., O'Grady, L. F., Macy, D. J., Mills, S. L., Epstein, A. J., Peng, J.-S., and McGahan, J. P. (1987). Treatment of a patient with B cell lymphoma by 1-131 LYM-1 monoclonal antibodies. *Int. J. Biol. Markers 2*: 49–53.

138. Hellman, S. (1985). Iodine 131 antiferritin, a new treatment modality in hepatoma: A radiation therapy oncology group study (Editorial). *J. Clin. Oncol. 3*: 1569.

139. Order, S. E., Stilwagon, G. B., Klein, J. L., Leichner, P. K., Sigelman, S. S., Fishman, E. K., Ettinger, D. S., Haulk, T., Kopher, K., Finney, K., Surdyke, M., Self, S., and Leibel, S. (1985). Iodine 131 antiferritin, a new treatment modality in hepatoma: A radiation therapy oncology group study. *J. Clin. Oncol. 3*: 1573–1582.

140. International Symposium on Labeled and Unlabeled Antibody in Cancer Diagnosis and Therapy. (1987). *NCI Monogr. 3*: 1–167.

141. Msirikale, J. S., Klein, J. L., Schroeder, J., and Order, S. E. Radiation enhancement of radiolabeled antibody deposition in tumors. *Int. J. Radiat. Oncol. Biol. Phys.* In press.

142. Sitzmann, J. V., Order, S. E., Klein, J. L., Leichner, P. K., Fishman, E. K., and Smith, G. W. Conversion by new treatment modalities of non-resectable to resectable hepatocellular cancer. *J. Clin. Oncol.* In press.

143. Yeh, M-Y., Hellström, I., and Hellström, K. E. (1981). Clonal variation in expression of a human melanoma antigen defined by a monoclonal antibody. *J. Immunol. 126*: 1312-1317.

144. Albino, A. P., Lloyd, K. O., Houghton, A. N., Oettgen, H. F., and Old, L. J. (1981). Heterogeneity in surface antigen and glycoprotein expression of cell lines derived from different melanoma metastases of the same patient. Implications for the study of tumor antigens. *J. Exp. Med. 154*: 1764-1778.

145. Cillo, C., Mach, J. P., Schreyer, M., and Carrel, S. (1984). Antigenic heterogeneity of clones and subclones from human melanoma cell lines demonstrated by a panel of monoclonal antibodies and flow microfluoremetry analysis. *Int. J. Cancer 15*: 11-20.

146. Pastran, I., Willingham, M. C., and FitzGerald, J. P. (1986). Immunotoxins. *Cell 47*: 641-648.

147. Thorpe, P. E. (1985). Antibody carriers of cytotoxic agents in cancer therapy: A review. In *Monoclonal Antibodies '84: Biological and Clinical Applications*. Edited by A. Pinchera, G. Doria, F. Dammacco, and A. Bargellesi. Editrice Kurtis, s.r.l., pp. 475-506.

148. Vitetta, E. S., and Uhr, J. W. (1985). Immunotoxins. *Annu. Rev. Immunol. 3*: 197-212.

149. Schultz, G., Bumol, T. F., and Reisfeld, R. A. (1983). Monoclonal-directed effector cells selectively lyse human melanoma cells in vitro and in vivo. *Proc. Natl. Acad. Sci. USA 80*: 5407-5411.

150. Spitler, L. E., del Rio, M., Khentigan, A., Wedel, N. I., Brophy, N. A., Miller, L. L., Harkonen, W. S., Rosendorf, L. L., Lee, H. M., Mischak, R. P., Kawahata, R. T., Stoudemire, J. B., Fradkin, L. B., Bautista, E. E., and Scannon, P. J. (1987). Therapy of patients with melanoma using a monoclonal antimelanoma antibody-ricin A chain immunotoxin. *Cancer Res. 47*: 1717-1723.

151. Tsukada, I., Bishop, W. K., Hibe, N., Hirai, H., Hurwitz, E., and Sela, M. (1982). Effect of conjugates of daunomycin and antibodies to rat alpha-fetoprotein-producing tumor cells. *Proc. Natl. Acad. Sci. USA 79*: 621-625.

152. Braun, J., Fugiwara, K., Pollard, T. D., and Unanue, E. R. (1978). Two distinct mechanisms for redistribution of lymphocyte surface macromolecules. I. Relationship to cytoplasmic myosin. *J. Cell Biol. 79*: 409-418.

153. Old, L. J., Stockert, E., Boyse, E. A., and Kim, J. H. (1968). Antigenic modulation: Loss of TL antigen from cells exposed to TL antibody. Study of the phenomenon in vitro. *J. Exp. Med. 127*: 523-539.

154. Lavie, E., Hirschberg, D., Hellström, K. E., and Hellström, I. (1987). Pharmacological properties of drug-polymers and drug-L6 antibody in human carcinoma cell lines: Use of a pH-sensitive linker between the drug and biomolecules. *Proc. 78th Ann. Meet Am. Assoc. Cancer Res. 28*: 388.

155. Lavie, E., Hirschberg, D., Schreiber, G., Thor, K., Hill, L., Hellström, I., and Hellström, K. E. In vitro and in vivo evaluation of daunomycin-polyers and daunomycin-L6 conjugates: Use of pH sensitive linker between drug and biomolecule. Manuscript submitted.

156. Thistlethwaite, A. J., Leeper, D. B., Moylan, D. J., and Nerlinger, R. E. (1985). pH distribution in human tumors. *Int. J. Radiat. Oncol. Bio. Phys. 11*: 1647–1652.

157. Blattler, W. A., Kuenzi, B. S., Lambert, J. M., and Senter, P. D. (1985). New heterobifunctional protein cross-linking reagent that forms an acid-labile link. *Biochemistry 24*: 1517–1524.

158. Anasettie, C., Martin, P. J., June, C. H., Hellström, K. E., Ledbetter, J. A., Rabinovitch, P. S., Morishita, Y., Hellström, I., and Hansen, J. A. (1987). Induction of calcium flux and enhancement of cytolytic activity in NK cells by crosslinking of the sheep erythrocyte binding protein (CD2) and the Fc-receptor (CD16). *J. Immunol. 139*: 1772–1779.

159. Livingston, P. O., Natoli, E. J., Calves, M. J., Stockert, E., Oettgen, H. F., and Old, L. J. (1987). Vaccines containig purified GM2 ganglioside elicit GM2 antibodies in melanoma patients. *Proc. Natl. Acad. Sci. USA 84*: 2911–1915.

160. Mackett, M., Smith, G. L., and Moss, B. (1982). Vaccinia virus: A selectable eukaryotic cloning and expression vector. *Proc. Natl. Acad. Sci. USA 79*: 7415–7419.

161. Bennink, J. R., Yewdell, J. W., and Gerhard, W. (1982). A viral polymerase involved in recognition of influenza virus-infected cells by a cytotoxic T-cell clone. *Nature 311*: 578–579.

162. Earl, P. L., Moss, B., Morrison, R. P., Wehrly, K., Nishio, J., and Chesbro, B. (1986). T-lymphocyte priming and protection against Friend leukemia by vaccinia-retrovirus env gene recombinant. *Science 23*: 728–731.

163. Lathe, R., Kieny, M. P., Gerlinger, P., Clertant, P., Guizani, I., Cuzin, F., and Chambon, P. (1987). Tumour prevention and rejection with recombinant vaccinia. *Nature 326*: 878–880.

164. Hu, S.-L., Plowman, G. D., Sridhar, P., Stevenson, U. S., Brown, J. P., and Estin, C. D. (1988). Characterization of a recombinant vaccinia virus expressing human melanoma-associated antigen p97. *J. Virol. 62*: 176–180.

165. Zbar, B., Bernstein, I. D., Bartlett, G. L., Hanna, M. G., Jr., and Rapp, H. J. (1972). Immunotherapy of cancer: Regression of intradermal tumors and prevention of growth of lymph node metastases after intradermal injection of living *Mycobacterium bovis*. *J. Natl. Cancer Inst. 49*: 119–130.

166. Klein, E. (1968). Tumors of the skin. X. Immunotherapy of cutaneous and mucosal neoplasms. *N.Y. State J. Med. 68*: 900–911.

167. Fidler, I. J., and Poste, G. (1982). Macrophage-mediated destruction of malignant tumor cells and new strategies for the therapy of metastatic disease. *Springer Semin. Immunopathol. 5*: 161–172.

168. Greenberg, P. D., Kern, D. E., and Cheever, M. A. (1985). Therapy of disseminated murine leukemia with cyclophosphamide and immune Lyt-1+, 2– T cells. Tumor eradication does not require participation of cytolytic T cells. *J. Exp. Med.* *161*: 1122–1134.

169. zur Hausen, H. (1987). Papillomaviruses in human cancer. *Cancer 59*: 1692–1696.

170. Urbain, J., Slaoui, M., and Leo, O. (1982). Idiotypes, recurrent idiotypes and internal images. *Ann. Immunol.* *133D*: 179–189.

171. Rajewski, K., and Takemori, T. (1983). Genetics, expression, and function of idiotypes. *Ann. Rev. Immunol.* *1*: 569–607.

172. Lee, V. K., Hellström, K. E., and Nepom, G. T. (1986). Idiotypic interactions in immune responses to tumor-associated antigens. *Biochim. Biophys. Acta 865*: 127–139.

173. Hellström, K. E., Lee, V. K., Nelson, K. A., and Hellström, I. (1987). Induction and analysis of tumor immunity using anti-idiotypic antibodies. *Monogr. Allergy 22*: 212–221.

174. Nepom, G. T., and Hellström, K. E. (1987). Anti-idiotypic antibodies and the induction of specific tumor immunity. *Cancer Metasta. Rev. 6*: 487–501.

175. Forstrom, J. W., Nelson, K. A., Nepom, G. T., Hellström, I., and Hellström, K. E. (1983). Immunization to a syngeneic sarcoma by a monoclonal auto-anti-idiotypic antibody. *Nature 303*: 627–629.

176. Nelson, K. A., George, E., Swenson, C., Forstrom, J. W., and Hellström, K. E. (1987). Immunotherapy of murine sarcomas with auto-anti-idiotypic monoclonal antibodies which bind to tumor-specific T cells. *J. Immunol. 139*: 2110–2117.

177. Kennedy, R. C., Deesman, G. R., Butel, J. S., and Lanford, R. E. (1985). Suppression of in vivo tumor formation induced by Simian virus 40-transformed cells in mice receiving anti-idiotypic antibodies. *J. Exp. Med. 161*: 1432–1449.

178. Lee, V. K., Harriott, T. G., Kuchroo, V. K., Halliday, W. J., Hellström, I., and Hellström, K. E. (1985). Monoclonal anti-idiotype antibodies related to a murine oncofetal bladder tumor antigen induce specific cell-mediated tumor immunity. *Proc. Natl. Acad. Sci. USA 82*: 6286–6290.

179. Herlyn, D., Ross, A. H., Koprowski, H. (1986). Anti-idiotypic antibodies bear the internal image of a human tumor antigen. *Science 232*: 100–102.

180. Nelson, K., Cory, J., Hellström, I., and Hellström, K. E. (1981). T-T hybridoma product specifically suppresses tumor immunity. *Proc. Natl. Acad. Sci. USA 77*: 2866–2870.

181. Nelson, K., Hellström, I., and Hellström, K. E. (1985). Tumor antigen-specific suppressor factors made by T cell hybridomas. In *T-Cell Hybridomas*. Edited by M. J. Taussig. CRC Press, Boca Raton, Florida, pp. 129–138.

182. Hellström, I., Hellström, K. E., Rollins, N., Lee, V. K., Hudkins, K., and Nepom, G. T. (1985). Monoclonal antibodies to cell surface antigens

shared by chemically induced mouse bladder carcinomas. *Cancer Res.* *45*: 2210-2218.

183. Kuchroo, V. K., Lee, V. K., Hellström, I., Hellström, K. E., and Halliday, W. J. (1987). Tumor-specific idiotopes on suppressor factors and suppressor cells revealed by monoclonal anti-idiotype antobodies. *Cellular Immunol. 104*: 105-114.

184. Bansal, S. C., and Sjögren, H. O. (1971). Unblocking serum activity in vitro in the polyoma system may correlate with antitumour effects of antiserum in vivo. *Nature (New Biol.) 233*: 76-78.

185. Bansal, S. C., and Sjögren, H. O. (1972). Counteractions of the blocking of cell-mediated tumor immunity by inoculation of unblocking sera and splenectomy: immunotherapeutic effects on primary polyoma tumors in rats. *Int. J. Cancer 9*: 490-509.

186. Bansal, S. C., and Sjögren, H. O. (1973). Regression of polyoma tumor metastasis by combined unblocking and BCG treatment—correlation with induced alterations in tumor immunity status. *Int. J. Cancer 12*: 179-193.

187. Hellström, I., and Hellström, K. E. (1970). Colony inhibition studies on blocking and non-blocking serum effect on cellular immunity to Moloney sarcomas. *Int. J. Cancer 5*: 195-201.

188. Hellström, K. E., Hellström, I., and Nepom, J. T. (1977). Specific blocking factors—are they important? *Biophys. Biochim. Acta Rev. Cancer 473*: 121-148.

189. Nepom, J. T., Hellström, I., and Hellström, K. E. (1977). Antigen-specific purification of blocking factors from sera of mice with chemically induced tumors. *Proc. Natl. Acad. Sci. USA 74*: 4605-4609.

190. Horn, L., and Horn, H. L. (1971). An immunological approach to the therapy of cancer? *Lancet ii*: 466-469.

191. Hellström, I., and Hellström, K. E. (1971). Some aspects of human tumor immunity and their possible implications for tumor prevention and therapy. In *Frontiers in Radiation Therapy and Oncology*. Karger, Basel, Chap. 7, pp. 3-15.

192. Wright, P. W., Hellström, K. E., Hellström, I., and Bernstein, I. (1976). Serotherapy of malignant disease. Symposium on immunotherapy of malignant disease. In *The Medical Clinics of North America*. Edited by D. Holmes. W. B. Saunders Co., Philadelphia, pp. 607-622.

193. Senter, P. D., Saulnier, M. G., Schreiber, G. J., Hirschberg, D. L., Brown, J. P., Hellström, I., and Hellström, K. E. (1988). Antitumor effects of antibody-alkaline phosphatase conjugates in combination with etoposide phosphate. *Proc. Natl. Acad. Sci. USA, 85*: 4842-4846.

2

Biochemical Engineering of Immunotoxins for Ex Vivo Bone Marrow Transplantation and In Vivo Leukemia Treatment

PIERRE CARAYON, PIERRE CASELLAS, and F. K. JANSEN
Sanofi Recherche, Montpellier, France

I. INTRODUCTION

Monoclonal antibodies reacting with human malignant cells offer new potential for tumor therapy. To date, treatment of cancer with monoclonal antibodies in vivo has not been very beneficial, probably due to a weak cytotoxic effect. In order to make these reagents more cytotoxic, immunotoxins can be made by linking powerful toxins such as ricin or its cytotoxic subunit to monoclonal antibodies (1).

Ricin is a potent toxin which is extracted from the castor bean. It contains two chains which have different functions. The B chain binds to galactose residues on the cell surface. After transfer into the cytosol of a cell, the A chain acts on the 60S ribosome subunits and inhibits protein synthesis (2). The basic concept of therapy with immunotoxin is to direct the A chain against specific target cells, which may be cancer cells, using a monoclonal antibody.

With the collaboration of H. Blythman, C. Bouloux, B. Bourrie, X. Canat, J. M. Derocq, D. Dussossoy, O. Gros, P. Gros, G. Laurent, G. Richer, and H. Vidal.

This chapter deals with the different methods used to prepare immunotoxins using either whole immunoglobulins or antigen-binding fragments thereof. The A chain can be linked to the antibody by several pathways. The activity of these immunotoxins in vitro will be described, followed by presentation of results obtained in ex vivo graft purging prior to allogeneic bone marrow transplantation, and on in vivo treatment of human B-cell chronic lymphocytic leukemia (B-CLL). Finally, we will present the latest information on research carried out in the lab designed to improve the efficacy of the immunotoxins in vivo.

II. BIOCHEMICAL ASPECTS OF IMMUNOTOXIN PREPARATION

A. A-Chain Preparation

Ricin is first purified by affinity chromatography on galactose-containing matrices, such as agarose gels. After dissociation with 5% mercaptoethanol, the A chain is separated from the B chain by two-step ion-exchange chromatography, carried out on agarose gels in order to increase the B chain retention by affinity to galactose residues on agarose. Immunopurification on Sepharose-bound purified goat antibodies raised against the B chain, yields an A chain preparation with less than 1/10,000 B-chain contamination.

B. Coupling of the A Chain to the Antibody

1. Disulfide Bridge

Two steps are necessary to couple the A chain to the monoclonal antibody; in the conventional design of immunotoxins, these steps are:

1. Heterobifunctional reagent SPDP (N-succinimidyl 3-(2-pyridyldithio)-propionate) reacts with the monoclonal antibody introducing two to four activated disulfide groups per molecule of antibody (Reaction 1).

Reaction 1

2. The modified monoclonal antibody is then mixed with an excess of A chain which reacts via its free sulphydryl group (Reaction 2).

A-SH + (pyridyl)-S—S—CH$_2$—CH$_2$—$\overset{\overset{\text{O}}{\|}}{\text{C}}$—NH-**Ab** ⟶

A chain   Activated MAb

A—S—S—CH$_2$—CH$_2$—$\overset{\overset{\text{O}}{\|}}{\text{C}}$—NH-**Ab** + (pyridine-thione)

Reaction 2   Immunotoxin

The conjugate is separated from unconjugated A chain on a Sephadex G200 column. In general, the final substitution ratio is 1.5 to 2 moles of A-chain per mole of immunoglobulin. The biological properties of the monoclonal antibody and of the A chain remain intact in the conjugate (3).

2. Thioether Bridge

In this case the disulfide bridge is replaced by a thioether bridge using, for example, the bifunctional coupling reagent, 6-maleimidocaproic acid (activated by a water-soluble carbodiimide) instead of SPDP.

3. Linkages Involving Different A-Chain Amino Acids

In order to study different possibilities of linking the A chain to the monoclonal antibodies, functions other than the natural thiol of the A chain can be used.

The thiol groups of the A chain must first be irreversibly blocked with an excess of N-ethylmaleimide after treatment with β-mercaptoethanol. The generation of artificially introduced thiol groups is then obtained using either S-acetyl mercaptosuccinic anhydride (SAMSA) for linkage to amino groups, or cystamine in the presence of the carbodiimide EDC for linkage to carboxyl groups (followed by reductive splitting of the disulfide bound of the coupled cystamine residues), or the imidazolide of 2-pyridyldithiopropionic acid for linkage to tyrosine residues (Reaction 3).

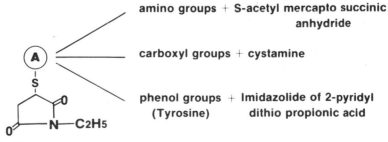

amino groups + S-acetyl mercapto succinic anhydride

carboxyl groups + cystamine

phenol groups + Imidazolide of 2-pyridyl (Tyrosine)   dithio propionic acid

Reaction 3

The A-chain can then be linked to the anti-CD5 T101 monoclonal antibody via a disulfide or a thioether bridge.

Acellular tests on rat liver microsomes permit the evaluation of the enzymatic activity of the A chain after these modifications. Only the modification on tyrosine residues decreases the enzymatic activity of the A chain by a factor of 3. The two other modifications on amino and carboxyl groups do not show any really significant decrease in activity.

II. ACTIVITY OF IMMUNOTOXINS IN VITRO

A. Immunotoxins Involving Coupling by Various Amino Acids of the A Chain

Before analyzing the cellular activities of these different immunotoxins, we present two methods currently used to evaluate their toxicity in vitro:

A protein synthesis inhibition assay measuring $[^{14}C]$ leucine incorporation into the cells after treatment with immunotoxins (4).

A colony inhibition assay in which cells are seeded in Petri dishes on agar to measure the proliferation of clonogenic tumor cells still viable after treatment (5).

The activities of ricin and of the immunotoxin directed against the Thy 1.2 differentiation antigen in the protein synthesis inhibition assay on the WEHI-7 cell line are presented in Figure 1. As shown in this figure, the A-chain molar concentration necessary to obtain 50% inhibition of protein synthesis (IC_{50}) is $2.6 \ 10^{-10} M$ for anti-Thy 1.2 immunotoxin and $9.1 \ 10^{-7} M$ for A chain alone. The factor of specificity is graphically represented by an arrow. The tail corresponds to the IC_{50} of free A chain and the head to IC_{50} of the immunotoxin. The factor of specificity for this anti-Thy 1.2 immunotoxin is 4000.

T101-A-chain immunotoxin directed against the human T-cell antigen CD5 present on lymphoblastoid CEM cell line was used as a model to investigate the influence of A-chain amino acids involved in the coupling to the antibody and the influence of the linkage (disulfide or thiother) (Table 1). Since the classical T101-immunotoxin, in which the natural thiol of the A chain is involved is only active in the presence of enhancers such as ammonium chloride or monensin, the activity of the above T101 immunotoxins was also tested in the presence of these enhancers.

The disulfide bridge is always more efficient than the thioether bridge in all kinds of linkages of the A chain to the monoclonal antibody (Table 1), at least when the antibody moiety is the T101 monoclonal antibody. Because the disulfide bond can be reversibly split under physiological conditions, in contrast

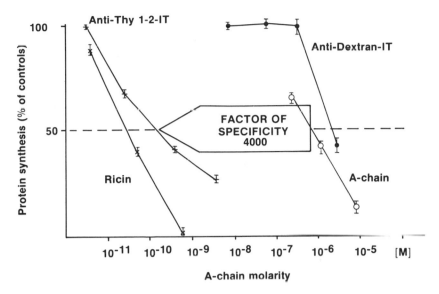

Figure 1 Activity of the anti-Thy 1.2 immunotoxin on WEHI-7 cell line. WEHI-7 cells were incubated with ricin (x———x) or with the specific anti-Thy 1.2 immunotoxin (+———+) or with nonrelevant toxins such as anti-dextran immunotoxin (●———●) or ricin A chain alone (o———o), at various doses, over 16 h. [^{14}C]leucine incorporation allows the A chain molarity (abscissa axis) necessary to inhibit 50% of protein synthesis (IC_{50}) into the cells (ordinate axis) to be determined. The factor of specificity is the ratio between the IC_{50} of the relevant anti-Thy 1.2 immunotoxin and that of free A chain alone.

to the thioether bridge, this may suggest that good immunotoxin activity requires an A chain which can be easily cleaved from the monoclonal antibody.

With respect to the different amino acids involved in the coupling, immunotoxins assembled with A chains modified on the carboxylic groups are as efficient as those assembled with the natural thiol of the A chain. In the presence of monensin as enhancer, the efficacy of immunotoxins constructed with A chains modified on amino or phenol groups decreases by factors of 3 and 30, respectively. The disulfide bridge was therefore considered the more appropriate to assemble all the immunotoxins.

B. Immunotoxins Containing Fragments of Monoclonal Antibodies

Coupling of the A chain using different amino acids did not improve the activity of immunotoxins, therefore, studies were carried out to see whether immuno-

Table 1 Influence of the A Chain Amino Acid Linkage Variations on the Cellular Activity of the Anti-CD5 T101 Immunotoxin

Groups involved in the coupling to the monoclonal antibody		Cellular activity on CEM cells (IC_{50}) (M)	
		Disulfide	Thioether
SH	NH_4Cl	$1.6 \times 10{-}12$	$5 \times 10{-}11$
	Monensin	$4.3 \times 10{-}14$	$1.0 \times 10{-}12$
COOH	NH_4Cl	$2 \times 10{-}12$	$2 \times 10{-}11$
	Monensin	Not determined	Not determined
NH_2	NH_4Cl	$1.6 \times 10{-}11$	Not determined
	Monensin	$1.0 \times 10{-}13$	$3.3 \times 10{-}12$
Phenol	NH_4Cl	Not determined	Not determined
	Monensin	$1.2 \times 10{-}12$	$3.0 \times 10{-}11$

toxins constructed with fragments of the T101 monoclonal antibody, obtained after papain or pepsin treatment, were more active on CEM cell line. Figure 2 shows an advantage of fragment immunotoxins in kinetics of protein synthesis inhibition, at the doses where all the target antigen is covered. The time necessary to reduce 90% of protein synthesis is obtained within 24 hours with Fab immunotoxin, within 34 hours with F(ab')2 immunotoxin, and within 60 hours with whole IgG immunotoxin.

The monovalent F(ab) immunotoxin could possibly follow a different intracellular pathway responsible for a better toxicity. However, the kinetics of cytoreduction of the bivalent F(ab')2 immunotoxin is also faster than with whole IgG immunotoxin. This suggests that the size of the carrier is probably important in the activity of the A chain.

C. Improvement of Cytotoxic Activity of Immunotoxins by Enhancers

Higher cytotoxicity of immunotoxins can be achieved in the presence of lysosomotropic amines such as ammonium chloride (NH_4Cl), or carboxylic ionophores such as monensin (6,7). How these agents enhance this activity is still

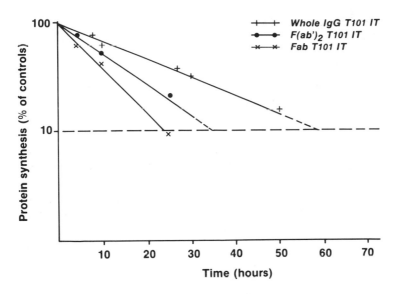

Figure 2 Kinetics of protein synthesis inhibition induced by T101 fragment immunotoxins. CEM cells were incubated with whole or fragment T101 immunotoxins at $10^{-8} M$ in A chain for various periods of time. The time necessary to reduce 90% of protein synthesis into the cells was 24 h for the Fab immunotoxin (x———x), 34 h for the F(ab')2 immunotoxin (•———•), and 60 h for the whole Ig G immunotoxin (+———+).

unknown. The IC_{50} values obtained with the T101 immunotoxin without enhancer, with NH_4Cl or monensin are, respectively, $2.10^{-9} M$, $3.10^{-13} M$, and $4.10^{-14} M$. In the presence of monensin, the IC_{50} value corresponds to as few as 10 molecules of T101 immunotoxin bound per cell. This has a great implication in the case of tumor cells with very low antigen density.

A dose of immunotoxin, where all the target antigen is covered, has been used to evaluate the cytotoxicity of immunotoxins on CEM cell line in a clonogenic assay. The cytotoxicity of the whole IgG T101 immunotoxin corresponds to one log cytoreduction, whereas a cytoreduction of 3 logs is observed with either fragment immunotoxins. In the presence of 10 mM NH_4Cl, the high sensitivity of the method does not permit to distinguish between fragment and whole IgG immunotoxins, since a cytoreduction higher than 6 logs is observed in each case (8).

IV. THERAPEUTIC APPLICATIONS OF IMMUNOTOXINS

A. Ex Vivo Use of Anti-CD5 Immunotoxins

To reduce the number of T lymphocytes in allogeneic bone marrow before its transplantation into compatible recipients, the first clinical trials were carried out using the whole IgG T101 immunotoxin. These trials were not conclusive. Since no reproducible cytoreduction of the T lymphocytes could be obtained in clinical conditions, a few treated patients presented severe acute graft-versus-host disease (GvHD). However, samples of the same donor bone marrow studied according to our routine laboratory methodology reproducibly conducted to 2 to 3 log cytoreduction. In an attempt to explain this discrepancy, various parameters were investigated, such as cell concentration, percentage of human serum albumin, purification of leukocytes, and pH. It was demonstrated that the active form of NH_4Cl, which enhances the immunotoxin efficacy, is the free base ammonia. This species rapidly diffuses across the cell membrane, but its concentration is highly dependent on the pH. At physiological pH, very little ammonia is available for the cells, therefore, in the presence of NH_4Cl, no cytoreduction is observed with whole IgG T101 immunotoxin. The level of cytoreduction increases as pH rises above 7.5. With Fab T101 immunotoxin, throughout the pH range 6.5–8.0 NH_4Cl leads to a much higher and less pH-dependent cytoreduction (Fig. 3) (9).

In the first clinical trials, bone marrow was generally collected and processed in the presence of citric acid as an anticoagulant, which led to pH values of 7.0 or even less. In subsequent clinical trials with Fab T101 immunotoxin, only heparin was used as an anticoagulant and the pH was raised and maintained at 7.8 using THAM acetate. Results obtained for cytoreduction in clinical conditions using this vehicle were similar to experimental data; the treated bone marrow lost more than 2 logs of T cells. Such T-cell depletion reduced the incidence of GvHD significantly. Among the first 38 patients treated according to the new protocol, only one developed grade II GvHD and no grade III or IV cases were experienced. However, bone marrow rejections (16%) were observed (10). This problem has also been observed with all other methods of T-cell depletion proposed, mainly using monoclonal antibodies plus complement. Modifications of the chemoradiotherapy conditioning regimens and of the conventional chemotherapy used to prevent GvHD may be able to circumvent these problems.

B. In Vivo Use of ITs

The CD5 antigen is present on T cells as well as on some malignant B cells, mainly in cases of chronic lymphocytic leukemia (B-CLL) (11). A patient with a B-CLL was therefore treated with whole IgG-T101 immunotoxin by intravenous injections over three consecutive days, at a daily dose of 25 mg.

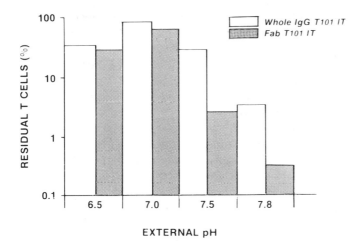

Figure 3 pH-dependence of whole or fragment T101 immunotoxins in the
presence of NH_4 Cl. Bone marrow mononuclear cells separated on gradient
density were treated with whole T101 immunotoxin (black column) or Fab-
T101 immunotoxin (stippled column) at $10^{-8}M$ in A chain, for 2 h in the
presence of 10 mM NH_4 Cl at various pH values. Mature T-cell cytoreduction was
evaluated by FACS analysis using a cocktail of fluorescent anti-T monoclonal
antibodies after immunotoxin-treated or nontreated samples had been cultivated for 3 days in the presence of phytohemagglutinin (PHA) and interleukin-2.

The aim of this pilot study was to assess clinical tolerability, to evaluate in
vivo binding of the immunotoxin onto target cells, and to follow its modulation
and pharmacokinetics in plasma.

Clinical efficacy was evaluated by the leukemic cell count in the peripheral
blood. A 40% decrease in the lymphocyte count, which remained stable over
two weeks, was observed. Although this effect was unusually long lasting, the
possibility could not be ruled out that it was partially due to the T101 moiety
itself, and not to the immunotoxin. Nevertheless, the administration of 75 mg of
T101 immunotoxin was perfectly well tolerated.

With respect to the binding of T101 immunotoxin to the leukemic cells, in
vivo complete saturation of cell surface antigens was obtained after a 2 h infusion. The target antigen and the immunotoxin gradually disappeared from the
cell surface. The peripheral lymphoblast count showed an immediate drop and
returned rapidly to initial values. The target antigen had reappeared at the cell
surface 24 h later (12).

T101 immunotoxin saturated all antigens present on target cells, but its
plasma level decreased 20-fold within 6 h after the end of perfusion. This rapid

clearance is hardly consistent with an efficient in vivo treatment, which requires high levels of immunotoxin in the blood and the extracellular compartments over a long period of time. Why was the clearance of the immunotoxin so rapid? The pharmacokinetics of the immunotoxin, the A chain, and the monoclonal antibody were compared in rabbits. The immunotoxin concentration as well as that of free A chain rapidly decreased in the plasma by three logs within a few hours, while the monoclonal antibody concentration declined at a much slower pace. The poor pharmacokinetics of the A chain can be explained by its glyco-protein nature. As shown in our own and other laboratories (13-15), the terminal mannose residues of its carbohydrate component are trapped by the Kupffer cells of the liver which present receptors to mannose. Administration of yeast mannan (a polymer of mannose), known to block plasma clearance of glycoproteins by blocking the mannose receptors of the liver, dramatically de-creases the clearance of ricin A chain and of the immunotoxins.

Alternatively, a partial chemical deglycosylation of the A chain was achieved using periodate oxidation. In rabbits, the pharmacokinetics of an immunotoxin with modified A chain was much improved, compared with that of the corres-ponding unmodified A-chain immunotoxin, without altering its potent cyto-toxic properties. Thus, a 350 times higher plasma level was obtained 24 h after administration.

The in vivo treatment of a B-CLL patient raised another problem of com-parable concern as that regarding the pharmacokinetics of the immunotoxins. This concerned the inefficient cell killing activity even when all target antigens had been saturated with immunotoxin. In clonogenic tests on CEM cells in vitro, this problem is overcome by the use of enhancers such as ammonium chloride or monensin (6). The concentrations of NH_4Cl necessary to activate immuno-toxins in vivo are highly toxic and unrealistic. Potentially, monensin could be used in vivo at safe concentrations, but with two major drawbacks: it is not hydrosoluble and its plasma half life is extremely short, less than 10 minutes, so that the necessary concentrations for the enhancement of immunotoxins in vivo cannot be obtained. However, when monensin was linked to human serum albumin (HSA), it became more hydrosoluble, its pharmacokinetic properties improved considerably in mouse experiments, and its enhancing properties were not lost. In these experiments, the plasma concentration of monensin as a bio-logically effective immunotoxin enhancer maintained higher levels than the minimum concentration necessary for in vitro enhancement for a period of sev-eral hours (16).

To demonstrate the capacity of HSA-monensin to enhance immunotoxins in vivo, we chose a murine lymphoma model in which only the T2 cancer cells grafted bore the Thy 1.2 antigen. The intravenous injection of T2 cells was followed one day later by the intravenous injection of HSA–monensin mixed with anti-Thy 1.2 immunotoxin, at doses at which neither product taken alone had any effect. All mice of the group treated with the immunotoxin associated to HSA-monensin survived for over 150 days. Mice treated with HSA-monensin or immunotoxin alone had the same mortality profile as the control group (16). In conclusion, future research needs to focus on the following points in order to make immunotoxins viable agents for cancer treatment in vivo:

The development of immunotoxins with deglycosylated A chain
The optimization of cell killing efficacy of immunotoxins in vivo with appropriate activators (HSA-monensin, chloroquine, etc.)
The search for new monoclonal antibody carriers in order to assemble immunotoxins directed against different types of leukemia or solid tumors.

Regarding this last point, intracavitary cancers such as ovarian carcinoma or bladder cancer, seem to present easier models for studies to be conducted near future because high doses of immunotoxins and enhancing agents can be administered in situ (17,18). If the in vivo enhancement of immunotoxins could be attained, a therapeutic tool complementary to classical cancer therapy could be envisaged with the particular aim of killing small metastases.

ACKNOWLEDGMENT

We thank Dr. C. Bouloux for reviewing the English translation of this work and A. Garcia for typing the manuscript.

REFERENCES

1. Jansen F. K., Blythman H. E., Carriere D., Casellas, P., Gros O., Gros P., Laurent J. C., Paolucci F., Pau B., Poncelet P., Richer G., Vidal H., and Voisin G. A. (1982). Immunotoxins hybrid molecules combining high specificity and potent cytotoxicity. *Immunol. Rev. 62*:185–216.
2. Olsnes S, Refsnes K., and Pihl A. (1974). Mechanism of action of the toxic lectins abrin and ricin. *Nature 249*:627–631.
3. Gros O., Gros P., Jansen F. K., and Vidal H. (1985). Biochemical aspects of immunotoxin preparation. *J. Immunol. Meth. 81*:283–297.
4. Jansen F. K., Blythman H. E., Carriere D., Casellas P., Diaz J., Gros P., Hennequin J. R., Paolucci F., Pau B., Poncelet P., Richer G., Salhi S. L., Vidal H., and Voisin G. A. (1980). High specific cytotoxicity of antibody-toxin hybrid molecules (immunotoxins) for target cells. *Immunol. Lett. 2*:97–102.
5. Jansen F. K., Poncelet P., Roncucci R., Vidal H., and Hellstrom K. E. (1982). Human melanoma cells can be killed in vitro by an immunotoxin specific for melanoma-associated p97. *Int. J. Cancer 30*:437–443.

6. Casellas P., Bourrie B. J. P., Gros P., and Jansen F. K. (1984). Kinetics of cytotoxicity induced by immunotoxin Enhancement by lysosomotropic amines and carboxylic ionophores. *J. Biol. Chem. 259*:9359–9364.

7. Raso V., and Lawrence J. (1984). Carboxylic ionophores enhance the cytotoxic potency of ligand and antibody delivered Ricin A-chain. *J. Exp. Med. 160*:1234–1240.

8. Derocq J. M., Casellas P., Laurent G., Ravel S., Vidal H., and Jansen F. K. Comparison of cytotoxic potency of T101 Fab F(ab')2 and whole IgG immunotoxins. Submitted for publication.

9. Casellas P., Ravel S., Bourri B. J. P., Derocq J. M., Jansen F. K., Laurent G., and Gros P. Entry of T101-ricin A-chain immunotoxin into human T-lymphocytes. Submitted for publication.

10. Laurent G., Maraninchi D., Gluckman E., Vernant J. P., Derocq J. M., Gaspard M. M., Rio B., Michalet M., Reiffers J., Dreyfus F., Casellas P., Bouloux C., Schneider P., Blythman H. E., and Jansen F. K. Donor bone-marrow treatment with T101 Fab fragment-ricin A-chain immunotoxin prevents graft-versus-host disease. Submitted for publication.

11. Royston I., Majda J. A., Baird S. M., Meserve B. L., and Griffiths J. C. (1980). Human T-cell antigens defined by monoclonal antibodies the 65 000 dalton antigen of T-cells (T65) is also found on chronic lymphocytic leukemia cells bearing surface immunoglobulin. *J. Immunol. 125*:725–731.

12. Laurent G., Pris J., Farcet J. P., Carayon P., Blythman H. E., Casellas P., Poncelet P., and Jansen F. K. (1986). Effects of therapy with T101 ricin A-chain immunotoxin in two leukemia patients. *Blood 67*:1680–1687.

13. Bourrie B. J. P., Casellas P., Blythman H. E., and Jansen F. K. (1986). Study of the plasma clearance of antibody-ricin-A-chain immunotoxins. Evidence for specific recognition sites on the A-chain that mediate rapid clearance of the immunotoxins. *Eur. J. Biochem. 155*:1–10.

14. Blakey D. C., and Thorpe P. E. (1986). Effect of chemicaldeglycosylation on the in vivo fate of ricin A-chain. *Cancer Drug Del. 3*:189–196.

15. (1987). Effect of chemical deglycosylation of ricin A-chain on the in vivo fate and cytotoxic activity of an immunotoxin composed of ricin A-chain and anti-Thy 1.2 antibody. *Cancer Res. 47*:947–952.

16. Dussossoy D., Blythman H. E., Casellas P., and Jansen F. K. In vivo potentiation of A-chain immunotoxins with HSA-monensin suppresses mouse leukemia. Submitted for publication.

17. Fitzgerald D. J. P., Willigham M. C., and Pastan I. (1986). Antitumor effects of an immunotoxin made with *Pseudomonas* exotoxin in a nude mouse model of ovarian cancer. *Proc.Natl. Acad. Sci.USA 83*:6627–6630.

18. Fitzgerald D. J. P., Bjorn M. J., Ferris R. J., Winkelhake J. L., Frankel A. E., Hamilton T. C., Ozols R. F., Willigham M. C., and Pastan I. (1987). Antitumor activity of an immunotoxin in a nude mouse model of human ovarian cancer. *Cancer Res. 47*:1407–1410.

3

Monoclonal Antibody 791T/36 Immunoconjugates for Cancer Treatment

ROBERT W. BALDWIN
Cancer Research Campaign Laboratories, University of Nottingham, Nottingham, England

VERA S. BYERS
XOMA Corporation, Berkeley, California

I. INTRODUCTION

Immunoconjugates constructed with antibodies reacting with human tumor-associated antigens are gaining in importance with regard to their use for cancer treatment (1). Chemoimmunoconjugates in which cytotoxic drugs are covalently linked to antibody have been prepared, the objective being to selectively deliver drug to tumor deposits and reduce normal tissue toxicity (1–3). Immunotoxins containing highly toxic plant and bacterial toxins covalently linked to antibody have also been synthesized (1). In this approach it is envisaged that the selective antibody targeting of toxin molecules will permit the administration of products which are too cytotoxic to be given in unconjugated form.

Monoclonal antibodies selected for the construction of covalently linked cytotoxic conjugates should react specifically with tumor cells or at least show only minimal reactivity with normal tissues. This is important since antibody reactivity with normal tissues or cells such as hematopoietic stem cells will be translated in vivo into toxicity.

For effective delivery of the cytotoxic moiety to the cell, the immunocon-jugate must be efficiently internalized into the intracellular compartment follow-ing binding to tumor cell surface antigens. This will reflect a number of separate but interrelated events, including the kinetics of association and dissociation of the antibody binding to tumor antigen and the efficiency of immunoconjugate internalization.

II. MONOCLONAL ANTIBODY 791T/36

Monoclonal antibody 791T/36 is produced by a hybridoma obtained by fusion of splenocytes from a mouse immunized against cells of a human osteogenic sarcoma cell line 791T and murine myeloma P3NSI (4). The antibody reacts with osteogenic sarcoma cells derived from cultured cell lines (5) and also with primary and metastatic osteogenic sarcomas (6). Reactivity is not confined to sarcomas since 791T/36 antibody also binds to cells derived from other tumor cell lines (5). More relevantly for clinical applications, 791T/36 binds to target cells derived from primary and metastatic colorectal carcinomas (7) and to ovarian carcinomas (Durrant et al., unpublished data). This has been investi-gated using an indirect immunofluorescence flow cytometry assay. Tumor cells were prepared from surgical specimens of tumor using a collagenase disaggrega-tion procedure and reacted with antibody 791T/36. Following treatment with fluorescein isothiocyanate (FITC)-labeled rabbit anti-mouse immunoglobulin, cells were analyzed by flow cytometry. Analysis was restricted to the size range of malignant cells by appropriate forward angle scatter gating, and control studies indicated that by these procedures there was approximately 20% contam-ination of tumor cell preparations with lymphocytes and stromal cells. In one series of studies, with target cells derived from 49 colorectal carcinomas, two-thirds showed adequate reactivity with antibody 791T/36 (7). Furthermore, tar-get cells derived from lymph node and hepatic metastases as well as pelvic recurrences have been shown to react with this antibody (8). This is of consider-able importance because it is postulated that therapy with immunoconjugates will be aimed at treating metastatic or recurrent disease.

Considerable variation in the level of expression of the antigen recognized by 791T/36 antibody was observed and the factors contributing to this are being investigated. One factor is tumor ploidy, with aneuploid tumors having the higher level of antigen expression (7). Relevant to these studies, related investi-gations have indicated that prognosis is poorer in patient with aneuploid tumors. This suggests that tumor cells amenable to immunoconjugate cytotoxicity are those contributing to the malignant phenotype.

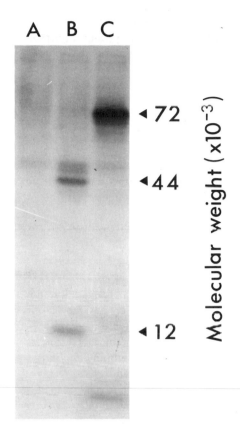

Figure 1 Radioimmunoprecipitation of 791T/36-defined antigen using 791T/36 monoclonal antibody and Sepharose-protein A. Immune precipitates, analyzed by SDS-PAGE and autoradiography, were prepared by the addition of antibodies and Sepharose protein A to lysates of ^{125}I-labeled 791T cells, as follows: *Lane A*: Normal mouse immunoglobulin; *Lane B*: Anti-HL-A – A, B, C, (shared determinant) clone W6/32; *Lane C*: 791T/32 monoclonal antibody.

III. IDENTIFICATION OF THE CELL ANTIGEN-BINDING 791T/36 ANTIBODY

Antibody 791T/36 reacts with a plasma membrane antigen on cultured human tumor cells. To determine the nature of this antigen osteogenic sarcoma 791T cells were surface labeled with ^{125}I, lysed and reacted with 791T/36 (9,10). The antigen reacting with 791T/36 migrated in sodium dodecyl sulfate-polyacrylamide gel electrophoresis (SDS-PAGE) gels with an apparent molecular weight of 72 kD. Both reduced and nonreduced SDS-PAGE analysis gave equivalent results indicating that the antigen is a monomeric cell surface product. Further biochemical analyses, including treatment with neuraminidase and proteolytic enzymes, analysis of product internally labeled with [^{3}H] glucosamine and purification by immunoadsorbent chromatography confirmed that the product binding to 791T/36 antibody is a 72 kD glycoprotein (Fig. 1). This gp72 product has been isolated from cultured tumor cell lines (sarcomas, carcinomas) which bind the antibody (10). The antigen on colon carcinomas 791T/36 antibody has been identified also as a 72 kD product (11). Thus immune complexes isolated from tumor extracts treated with [^{125}I] 791T/36 and analyzed by SDS-PAGE and autoradiography identified a 72 kD product together with two bands at 50 kD and 25 kD corresponding to those of the heavy and light chains of the 791T/36 antibody.

IV. LOCALIZATION OF MONOCLONAL ANTIBODY 791T/36 IN COLORECTAL AND OVARIAN CANCERS

Targeting of immunoconjugates containing cytotoxic agents depends upon the effective localization of the antibody moiety in the tumor. This has been established with 791T/36 antibody in a series of trials showing that ^{131}I and ^{111}In-labeled preparations localize in primary and metastatic colorectal cancers (12,13). In one prospective study carried out on 23 patients with a clinical suspicion of recurrence using ^{111}In-labeled 791T/36, 4 of 6 abdominal recurrences and 11 of 17 pelvic recurrences were detected, these results being in close agreement with computed tomography (CT) and x-ray evaluation (14,15). Assay of resected specimens from patients with colorectal cancer injected with [^{131}I]-791T/36 has also been used to demonstrate tumor localization (12,13). In this study, the ratio of ^{131}I radioactivity in tumor compared with adjacent 'normal' colonic tissue was 2.5:1 ± 1.1.

V. MONOCLONAL ANTIBODY 791T/36 IMMUNOCONJUGATES

Two approaches have been adopted in designing covalently linked conjugates of cytotoxic agents with monoclonal antibody 791T/36. In the first approach, cytotoxic drugs in clinical use have been conjugated to antibody either directly or through human serum albumin as a carrier to increase drug:antibody ratio (2,3). Drugs investigated for this purpose include methotrexate, daunomycin, and vindesine. The alternative approach has been to conjugate highly cytotoxic moieties which, because of their reactivity, cannot be administered in free form. This is exemplified by the construction of ricin A chain (RTA) immunoconjugates (4).

VI. METHOTREXATE-791T/36 ANTIBODY
CONJUGATES

Conjugates containing methotrexate (MTX) directly linked to antibody have
been prepared by incubating equimolar amounts of MTX, N-hydroxysuccinimide,
and dicyclohexyl carbodiimide for several hours. Substituted 791T/36 antibody
was then prepared by reacting the MTX ester with antibody to yield products
with an average molar substitution ratio in the range 2-5:1.

Conjugates have been synthesized also in which human serum albumin (HSA)
is employed as a drug carrier (16). Essentially MTX–HSA conjugates were prepared by reacting an excess of MTX and ethyl carbodiimide with HSA and then
removing polymeric products by size-exclusion chromatography (SEC). Iodo-
acetyl-substituted antibody was produced by reaction of antibody with a three-
to-fourfold molar excess of N-hydroxysuccinimidyl iodoacetate. The MTX-HSA
was treated with dithiothreitol to introduce a sulphydryl group and the product
reacted with iodoacetylated antibody. Following fractionation conjugates with
MTX:antibody ratios of the order of 30 to 40:1 were obtained (molecular
weight range up to 340 Ka).

VII. ANTIBODY REACTIVITY

Antibody binding properties of conjugates have been assessed by competition
at saturation with FITC-labeled unconjugated antibody for binding to antigen
bearing target tumor cells (17,18). In this procedure conjugate is mixed with
FITC-labeled 791T/36 antibody and the mixture reacted with 791T tumor cells
under conditions of antibody excess. The relative amounts of FITC-labeled antibody is measured by quantitative flow cytofluorimetry and mathematical procedures are used to facilitate interpretation of competition data in terms of
antibody binding activity (18). This then provides an assessment of antibody reactivity in MTX conjugates relative to that of unconjugated antibody. Using this
procedure conjugates containing up to 3 mol MTX/mol antibody retain 60 to
80% of antibody reactivity. Conjugates prepared following MTX-HSA linkage
to antibody retained approximately 40% of the reactivity of unsubstituted
antibody.

VIII. IN VITRO CYTOTOXICITY OF MTX-
791T/36 CONJUGATES

The in vitro cytotoxicity of MTX-antibody conjugates has been measured both
by a short-term cytotoxicity assay and by longer assay involving inhibition of
tumor cell colony formation (2,19). In the cytotoxicity assay, tumor cells were
incubated with a range of conjugates in microtiter plates for 24 to 48 h, and

Table 1 Cytotoxicity of Methotrexate-791T/36 Antibody Conjugates

Reagent	Cytotoxicity (IC_{50} ng/ml against osteogenic sarcoma (791T)
Direct conjugate	
MTX-791T/36 (MDC27)	204.0
MTX	6.6
MTX-791T/36 (MDC30)	178.0
MTX	6.0
MTX-791T/36 (MDC31)	70.8
MTX	12.6
HSA carrier conjugate	
MTX-HSA-791T/36 (MT5)	18.6
MTX	6.2
MTX-HSA-791T/36 (MT17)	2.4
MTX	4.8
MTX-HSA-791T/36 (MT18)	50.0
MTX	10.0

tumor cell survival determined by postincubation with [^{75}Se] selenomethionine (19). From the dose–response curves, the dose of methotrexate (free of conjugated) producing 50% inhibition of tumor cell survival (IC_{50}) was determined. Table 1 summarizes representative tests with MTX-conjugates compared with free MTX against 791T target cells. There was considerable variation in the reactivity of individual preparations, but in general conjugates produced with HSA carrier were more reactive. The sensitivity of target tumor cells also varied, one factor being the level of expression of the gp72 antigen reacting with 791T/36.

Table 2 Colony Inhibition Tests with Methotrexate-791T/36 Antibody Conjugates

Cell line	Antigen density[a]	IC_{50} (molarity)[b] 791T/36-HSA-MTX
791T	6×10^5	1.5×10^{-8}
788T	3×10^5	5.5×10^{-8}
T24	3×10^4	1.5×10^{-6}
Mel 2a	$< 5 \times 10^3$	$> 1.5 \times 10^{-5}$

[a]Mean number of antibody binding sites per cell.
[b]Expressed in terms of MTX content.

This is illustrated in Table 2 which summarizes colony inhibition tests with
MTX-HSA-791T/36 conjugates. Cell lines expressing the target antigen were
highly susceptible to the immunoconjugate (IC_{50} $1-6 \times 10^{-8}$ M MTX) compared to a 'weakly' antigenic line such as bladder carcinoma T24 (IC_{50} 1.5×10^{-6} M MTX).

IX. IN VIVO STUDIES

The therapeutic efficacy of MTX-HSA-791T/36 immunoconjugates compared
with free MTX has been assessed using the MTX-sensitive sarcoma 791T developing as xenografts in immunoderived mice (3). In these studies one treatment
protocol (twice weekly intraperitoneal injection for 5 weeks) demonstrated an
improved response with immunoconjugate compared with free drug. The T/C
ratio [tumor weights in treated:untreated (control) mice] with free MTX was
0.30 at a total drug dose of 60 mg/kg. Immunoconjugate produced at a T/C
ratio of 0.5 at 10–20 mg/kg and in one test almost complete suppression of

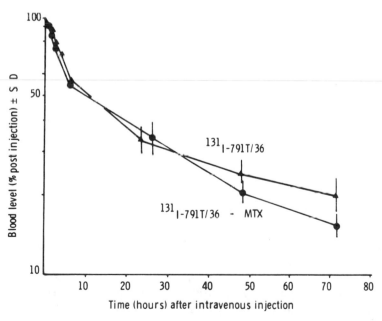

Figure 2   Kinetics of blood survival in BALB/c mice of [^{131}I]791T/36 antibody and [^{131}I](791T/36-methotrexate) conjugate. Points represent the mean
of samples from three mice after injection of 5 kBq of preparation.

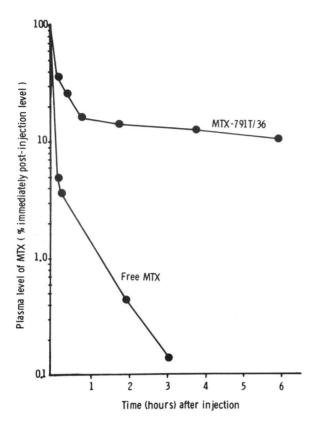

Figure 3 Kinetics of blood survival in mice of methotrexate injected free or as MTX-791T/36 monoclonal antibody conjugate. Mean of two mice/time point.

tumor growth was achieved with a total dose of MTX of 14 mg/kg in immunoconjugate form.

From the data generated over a large series of xenograft studies, it is evident that there is a considerable variation in the therapeutic response. One of the factors is thought to be the influence of the MTX residues on the biodistribution of the immunoconjugate (20).

The blood clearance of ^{131}I-labeled 791T/36 antibody in immunocompetent BALB/c mice is essentially biphasic, with an initial rapid clearance so that 40 to 50% of the injected dose is cleared within the first 5 h (Fig. 2). This is followed by a much slower elimination over the following 60 h with 10 to 20% of the injected dose still circulating after 70 h. Analysis of MTX-791T/36 immunoconjugates containing up to 3 mol MTX/mol antibody behave in a similar fashion (Fig. 2). The blood survival patterns of preparations containing 791T/36 antibody linked to HSA-MTX conjugate is markedly different. Thus biodistribution studies in normal BALB/c mice of conjugates containing 791T/36 antibody linked to [^{125}I] HSA-MTX showed that greater than 90% of the injected dose of radioactivity was removed from peripheral blood within 30 minutes of administration. This was principally due to rapid hepatic uptake of the MTX-HSA-791T/36 conjugate probably due to conjugate recognition by Kupffer cells.

Biodistribution studies have traditionally used MTX conjugates containing radioiodine-labeled antibody or human serum albumin (20). More recently, it has become possible to monitor plasma and tissue levels of methotrexate using a competitive radioimmunoassay (21) with a polyclonal antimethotrexate antiserum (Guildhay Antisera, Guildford, Surrey, England). These investigations are still ongoing, but they clearly show prolonged blood survival of MTX in normal BALB/c mice when injected as a direct conjugate with 791T/36 antibody. As illustrated in Figure 3, approximately 10% of the injected dose of MTX was present in plasma as antibody conjugate. In comparison, free MTX was rapidly eliminated over a 3 h period. Analysis of plasma and tissue levels of MTX in athymic mice bearing xenografts of tumor 791T demonstrate that the improved blood survival of MTX in antibody conjugate form leads to increased tumor deposition. Thus, in one series, the tumor MTX level (expressed as percent injected dose of MTX/g tissue) in mice treated with MTX-791T/36 was 10-50 times greater than in mice treated with free drug (20,22).

X. CLINICAL STUDIES

The blood survival of [^{131}I]-labeled 791T/36 antibody in patients with colorectal carcinoma has been determined as part of the immunoscintography studies (12, 13). The blood clearance of [^{131}I]-labeled antibody was biphasic, with an initial fall in blood levels of radioactivity over the first 24 h followed by a slower rate of clearance over the following 3 days (Fig. 4). Overall, the mean blood half life of antibody was 27 h. A total of 15 patients with colorectal cancer have been investigated following intravenous injection of [^{131}I]-labeled MTX-791T/36 conjugate. The blood survival of the radioiodine-labeled antibody component was closely similar to that of the unconjugated antibody (blood half life 30 h). These studies do not prove unequivocally that circulating antibody remained conjugated to MTX, although in vitro studies have established that these covalently linked conjugates in serum are stable for long periods of time. Further trials are now planned using the sensitive radioimmunoassay for methotrexate to determine the survival time in blood of the MTX conjugates.

Eleven of the patients treated with [^{131}I] MTX-791T/36 were examined by immunoscintigraphy. For this purpose patients were also injected with technetium-99m-labeled human [^{99m}Tc) serum albumin and [^{99m}Tc] sodium

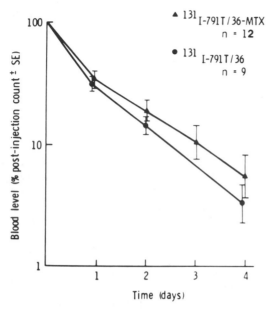

Figure 4 Kinetics of blood survival of [^{131}I] 791T/36 antibody and [^{131}I]-(791T/36-methotrexate) conjugate following intravenous injection to patients with colorectal cancer. Each received about 70 MBq of preparation.

pertechnetate to simulate the vascular and extravascular distribution of the antibody conjugate (23). Simultaneous ^{131}I and ^{99m}Tc images were recorded and image subtraction performed. Using these procedures, three of six colonic tumors and two of five rectal cancers were detected. The low detection rate of rectal tumors is influenced by free radioiodine in the bladder. In two of four patients with liver metastases, positive antibody images were obtained.

Because patients had been injected with radiolabeled MTX-791T/36 conjugate preoperatively, an assessment of radioactivity in tumor and normal adjacent colonic tissue was possible. The mean uptake of radioactivity in tumor compared to normal colonic tissue in 10 surgical specimens was 3.2:1, this being comparable to the localization of unconjugated antibody where tumor:normal colonic tissue ratios were 2.5:1 (12). Again these investigators are being extended and repeated to determine tissue levels of MTX.

XI. RICIN A CHAIN—791T/36 ANTIBODY CONJUGATES

Conjugates containing monoclonal antibody 791T/36 linked via a disulfide linkage to the A chain subunit of ricin toxin (from *Ricinus communis*) have

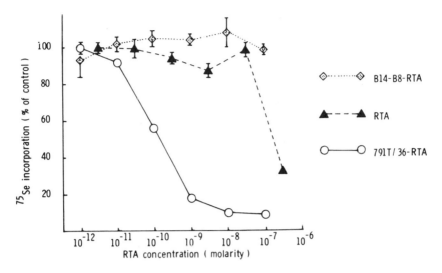

Figure 5 Cytotoxicity of 791T/36-RTA conjugate cells compared with that of free RTA and an irrelevant immunotoxin B14.B8-RTA: [^{75}Se] seleno-methionine incorporation assay (4).

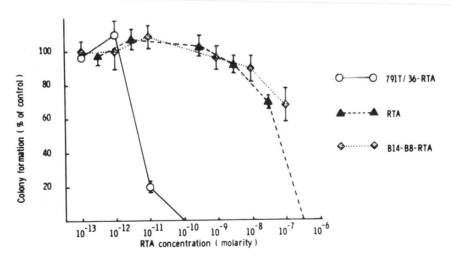

Figure 6 Colony inhibition assay of 791T/36-RTA cytotoxicity for 791T cells (4).

Table 3 Colony Inhibition Tests with RTA-791T/36 Antibody Conjugates

Cell line	Antigen density[a]	IC_{50} (molarity)[b] 791T/36-RTA
791T	6×10^5	1.4×10^{-10}
788T	3×10^5	1.6×10^{-10}
T24	3×10^4	2.2×10^{-9}
Mel 2a	$< 5 \times 10^3$	$> 10^{-6}$

[a]Mean number of antibody binding sites per cell.
[b]Expressed in terms of RTA content.

been synthesized (4,24). Analysis of antibody reactivity of the immunotoxins determined by the competitive flow cytometry assay described earlier with 791T target cells demonstrated that they retained between 60 and 80% of that of unconjugated antibody. Cytotoxicity of conjugate was assayed both by inhibition of [^{75}Se] selenomethionine into target cells and by their ability to inhibit tumor cell colony formation. Representative ^{75}Se cytotoxicity tests in Figure 5 indicate that 791T/36-RTA is at least 1000 times more cytotoxic for 791T cells than unconjugated RTA. Furthermore, an immunotoxin B14/B8-RTA, which does not bind to 791T cells, was essentially inactive in this system. The high cytotoxicity of 791T/36-RTA for 791T cells was even more clearly revealed by colony inhibition assays (Fig. 6). In this case the specific immunotoxin was about four orders of magnitude more cytotoxic than either free RTA or B14B8-RTA.

The specificity of the cytotoxicity of 791T/36-RTA was further explored against a panel of target cells where the level of gp72 antigen expression has been defined (Table 3). All of these target cells showed comparable susceptibility to free RTA, the concentration producing 50% inhibition of cell survival being 1.2 to 2.0×10^{-7} M. Cell lines having the highest density of gp72 antigen, such as sarcomas 791T and 788T, were susceptible to the immunotoxin (IC_{50} 1.4 and 1.6×10^{-10} M RTA). Cells expressing intermediate levels of the gp72 antigen (bladder carcinoma T24) were some tenfold less susceptible to the immunotoxin, and target cells with only threshold levels of gp72 antigens were insensitive.

These in vitro studies indicate that RTA conjugated to 791T/36 antibody yields a powerfully cytotoxic immunoconjugate.

XII. IN VIVO STUDIES

The efficacy of 791T/36-RTA immunotoxin has been demonstrated in extensive experiments in which growth of xenografts of human tumors expressing

Table 4 Inhibition of Growth of Tumor 791T Xenografts by XMMCO-791T RTA

Treatment Schedule		Mean tumor weights in treated/control groups (T/C)
Days	Total dose (mg/kg)	
20	100	0.30
15	75	0.30
10	50	0.36
5	25	0.25

gp72 antigen has been inhibited (24). This is illustrated by the experiments summarized in Table 4, where the influence of immunotoxin treatment has been assessed from the weights of tumor in treated (T) and control (C) groups at the termination of the experiment. Treatment of mice with immunotoxin (total dose 50 mg/kg) suppressed growth of tumor 791T (T/C 0.36), but free RTA was ineffective. Also treatment of another tumor, melanoma AAA232, did not produce a significant response.

Following from those initial investigations, a series of studies has been carried out to determine the most efficacious therapeutic procedure in terms of immunotoxin dose and treatment protocol. To be deemed reliable, these studies must take into account the biodistribution of immunotoxin, since following systemic administration the reactive species must have adequate blood survival to allow extravasation and penetration of the immunotoxin into the target tumor. This approach was selected as being relevant to subsequent clinical studies and no attempt was made to investigate intralesional injection of immunotoxin or cavity injection comparable to approaches being made with intraperitoneal tumors (25,26).

Pharmacokinetic studies with ricin and ricin A chain have shown that they are rapidly eliminated from blood with predominant localization in nonparenchymal hepatic cells (27). This pattern of organ distribution is due to the recognition of mannose-containing oligosaccharide side chains of ricin or the ricin A chain by specific cell surface receptors on hepatic Kupffer cells (28). Linking RTA to monoclonal antibody 791T/36 also markedly accelerated the removal of the conjugate from the blood when injected into normal BALB/c mice (Fig. 7) or athymic mice bearing tumor xenografts (29). This is due to the RTA moiety being taken up into the liver where the immunotoxin undergoes deconjugation.

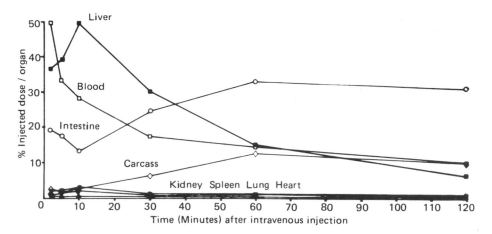

Figure 7 Organ distribution of ^{131}I radioactivity in normal BALB/c mice following injection of [^{131}I-RTA]-791T/36 conjugate (29).

Several groups have studied the interaction between mannose-containing oligosaccharides of RTA and mannose receptors on Kupffer cells in the liver (27,28,30), and various approaches are being investigated to circumvent this problem, including the construction of immunotoxins using RTA in which the terminal mannose groups on the oligosaccharides are reduced or chemically modified so as to prevent their recognition by Kupffer cells (27). Another approach has been to incorporate mannose-containing agents with the RTA immunotoxins in order to limit hepatic uptake. The effect of a range of 'mannose-containing' blockers has been examined with 791T/36-RTA (29). Glycoproteins and glycopeptides, including ovalbumin and ovomucoid as well as synthetic mannose-containing peptides such as a product containing mannose linked to lysyl-lysine (31), produced a marked inhibition of hepatic uptake. Mannosyl-lysine produced a fourfold reduction in the liver to blood ratio of radioactivity following injection of radiolabeled immunotoxin and this led to a considerable increase in blood survival of the product. Furthermore, deconjugation of immunotoxin occurs following hepatic uptake, therefore, the product retained in the peripheral blood was shown to be intact immunotoxin with the characteristics of the injected material. The incorporation of hepatic blocking agents has led to improved localization of immunotoxin in tumor xenografts, and it is anticipated that protocols utilizing these reagents will lead to improved therapeutic efficacy.

XIII. DISCUSSION

Investigations with monoclonal antibody 791T/36 have established that covalent linkage of cytotoxic agents yields immunoconjugates specifically cytotoxic for target cells expressing the antigen (gp72) recognized by the antibody. The in vitro cytotoxicity of immunoconjugates can be reproduced in vivo for treatment of human tumor xenografts, and based upon these studies, a phase I clinical trial is being conducted in patients with colorectal cancer (Byers et al. to be published). The preclinical investigations allow identification of various issues which are being addressed to facilitate further improvements in the design of immunoconjugates for cancer treatment.

Considering first the choice of cytotoxic agent, direct conjugation of methotrexate to antibody results in a substantial reduction of drug activity when compared with that of free drug. Thus in vitro cytotoxicity tests showed that the IC_{50} increased from around 5 to 10 ng/ml to 180 ng/ml and greater. This is similar to experiences with other drugs such as vindesine and daunomycin, where the reduction in cytotoxicity in the immunoconjugates was even greater (2,32,33), although overall this loss of drug activity is compensated for by the specificity of drug action imposed through the antibody moiety. In comparison, the effect was completely reversed with ricin A chain where antibody conjugation produces a 10^3 to 10^4-fold increase in cytotoxicity (4). This is because the toxin A chain is not readily internalized in the absence of the B chain. In contrast, antibody conjugation of cytotoxic drugs essentially abrogates their normal pathway for entry into a cell, this now depending upon mechanisms as yet not well understood, of antibody endocytosis. Two main types of endocytosis have been described, namely pinocytosis and receptor-mediated endocytosis (34,35). Pinocytosis, a constitutive uptake of soluble molecules, is concentration dependent, nonsaturable with uptake relatively slow and linear over a long time period (34). Receptor-mediated endocytosis, involving uptake via coated pits is rapid and efficient, cells taking up several times the number of molecules required to saturate cell surface receptors (35). Fluorescence analysis of the endocytosis of model conjugates constructed by conjugation of 791T/36 antibody to human serum albumin linked to tetramethylrhodamine (TRITC-HSA-791T/36) indicates that endocytosis probably occurs by pinocytosis with conjugates localizing within an acidic internal compartment of the tumor cell (36). It has also been estimated that as much as 50% of the cell-bound conjugate is endocytosed over a 4-h period. Although this rate of endocytosis is slower than that observed with receptor-mediated endocytosis, 791T/36 antibody conjugates are able to localize intracellularly without the need for potentiation.

Methods are being explored to improve drug delivery by monoclonal antibodies. Drug carrier systems are being developed, exemplified by the use of human serum albumin–methotrexate conjugates (16), which provides the means for coupling large amounts of drug to an antibody molecule. MTX-HSA-791T/36 conjugates are at least as, and sometimes more, cytotoxic than free drug. Earlier work demonstrated that excess of free 791T/36 antibody completely abrogated the in vitro cytotoxicity of the conjugate indicating that binding of the antibody moiety to the gp72 cell antigen was essential for cytotoxicity (37). Inhibitors of lysosomal acidity (ammonium chloride) and lysosomal proteases (leupeptin, pepstatin, chymotrypsin, and E64) also showed that lysosomal degradation was necessary for conjugate cytotoxicity and, in particular, thiol proteases were most active for the MTX conjugate (38). These observations, together with the work already referred to on the endocytosis of conjugates, indicate that internalization of conjugate mediated by the antibody moiety results in the intracellular release of methotrexate from the HSA-MTX component. The intracellular mechnisms yielding methotrexate in an active form are still not known, but these findings are important, indicating as they do that methotrexate is actively and efficiently transported into the cell when targeted as a MTX-HSA-791T/36 immunoconjugate.

Biodistribution studies with MTX-HSA-791T/36 conjugates have indicated that these conjugates need to be further refined to optimize their blood survival and hence delivery to target tissue. Investigations are ongoing to determine why this inadequacy persists since it is not thought to be only a feature of the increased molecular size when HSA carrier systems are used. Other factors thought to be important are the overall charge and hydrophobicity of the conjugates. One approach here is to design alternative drug carrier systems rather than depend on natural products such as protein and polysaccharides (dextran), and synthetic drug carrier systems are being evaluated.

From the investigations reported with several cytotoxic drugs, it is considered that products directly linked to antibody are unlikely to be of sufficient potency for therapeutic use. This has spurred the search for more potent cytotoxic agents such as aminopterin to replace methotrexate. It may also be possible to increase the amount of drug delivered to a cell by using combinations of antibodies which react with different epitopes.

Immunotoxins in which ricin chain is linked to monoclonal antibody 791T/36 are much more cytotoxic than the MTX conjugates when tested in vitro against target cells expressing the gp72 antigen. This in vitro cytotoxic potential has been translated in vivo to show that the immunotoxin suppresses growth of tumor xenografts including those established from colorectal cancers (24). On this basis, a phase I clinical trial in colorectal cancer has been set up (Byers et al. to be reported). Pharmacokinetic studies with 791T/36-RTA indicate again that improvements in the blood survival of the immunotoxin are desirable because of possibility for increased therapeutic potential. This potential can be realized using agents which specifically inhibit the uptake of immunotoxin by hepatic Kupffer cells (29). The next phase of these studies will examine the influence of those 'blocking agents' on the efficacy of immunotoxins against human tumor xenografts.

The efficiency of immunotoxin internalization into target cells is also a critical step in the cytotoxic response. With immunotoxins active against T leukemia cells and T lymphocytes, potentiators such as ammonium chloride or the carboxylic ionophore monensin are essential to yield a meaningful cytotoxic response (39). This is not the case with 791T/36-RTA immunotoxin because neither monensin or ammonium chloride have significantly increased its cytotoxicity for tumor target-cells. This further emphasizes the efficiency of the 791T/36 antibody molecule in intracellular transport of the cytotoxic moiety in immunotoxin.

REFERENCES

1. Baldwin, R. W., and Byers, V. S. (1987). Monoclonal antibodies and immunoconjugates for cancer treatment. *Cancer Chemother. Ann. 9*, 409–431.
2. Baldwin, R. W., Embleton, M. J., Gallego, J., Garnett, M., Pimm, M. V., and Price, M. R. (1986). Monoclonal antibody drug conjugates for cancer therapy. *Monoclonal Antibodies in Cancer: Advances in Diagnosis and Treatment.* Edited by J. Roth, Futura, Mt. Kisco, NY, Chap. 8, pp. 215–257.
3. Baldwin, R. W. (1987). Monoclonal antibody 791T/36: drug conjugates for cancer therapy. In *New Avenues in Developmental Cancer Chemotherapy.* Edited by Harrap and Connors. Academic Press, Inc., pp. 277–290.
4. Embleton, M. J., Byers, V. S., Lee, H. M., Scannon, P., Blackhall, N. W., and Baldwin, R. W. (1986). Sensitivity and selectivity of ricin toxin A chain —monoclonal antibody 791T/36 conjugates against human tumor cell lines. *Cancer Res. 46*:5524–5528.
5. Embleton, M. J., Gunn, B., Byers, V. S., and Baldwin, R. W. (1981). Antitumour reactions of monoclonal antibody against a human osteogenic sarcoma cell line. *Br. J. Cancer 43*:582–587.
6. Roth, J. A., Restropo, C., Scuderi, P., Baldwin, R. W., Reichert, C. M., and Hosoi, S. (1984). Analysis of antigenic expression of primary and autologous metastatic sarcomas using monoclonal antibodies. *Cancer Res. 44*:5320–5325.
7. Durrant, L. G., Robins, R. A., Armitage, N. C., Brown, A., Baldwin, R. W., and Hardcastle, J. D. (1986). Association of antigen expression and DNA ploidy in human colorectal tumors. *Cancer Res. 46*:3543–3549.
8. Ballantyne, K. C., Durrant, L. G., Armitage, N. C., Robins, R. A., Baldwin, R. W., and Hardcastle, J. D. (1986). Binding of a panel of monoclonal antibodies to primary and metastatic colorectal cancer. *Br. J. Cancer 54*:191.
9. Price, M. R., Campbell, D. G., Robins, R. A., Blecher, T. E., and Baldwin, R. W. (1984). Characteristics of the cell surface antigen, p72, associated with a variety of human tumours and mitogen stimulated T lymphoblasts. *FEBS Lett. 171*:31–35.

10. Campbell, D. G., Price, M. R., and Baldwin, R. W. (1984). Analysis of a human osteogenic sarcoma antigen and its expression on various human tumour cell lines. *Int. J. Cancer 34*:31–37.
11. Price, M. R., Pimm, M. V., Page, C. M., Armitage, N. C., Hardcastle, J. D., and Baldwin, R. W. (1984). Immunolocalization of the murine monoclonal antibody, 791T/36 within primary human colorectal carcinomas and identification of the target antigen. *Br. J. Cancer 49*:809–812.
12. Armitage, N. C., Perkins, A. C., Pimm, M. V., Farrands, P. A., Baldwin, R. W., and Hardcastle, J. D. (1984). The localisation of an anti-tumour monoclonal antibody (791T/36) in gastrointestinal tumours. *Br. J. Surg. 71*:407–412.
13. Armitage, N. C., Perkins, A. C., Pimm, M. V., Wastie, M. L., Baldwin, R. W., and Hardcastle, J. D. (1985). Imaging of primary and metastatic colorectal cancer using an ^{111}In-labelled antitumour monoclonal antibody (791T/36). *Nucl. Med. Commun. 6*:623–631.
14. Ballantyne, K. C., Perkins, A. C., Armitage, N. C., Pimm, M. V., Baldwin, R. W., and Hardcastle, J. D. (1986). Comparison of ^{131}I and ^{111}In-labelled monoclonal antibody 791T/36 in the detection of recurrent colorectal cancer. *Nucl. Med. Commun. 7*:309.
15. Perkins, A. C., Ballantyne, K. C., and Pimm, M. V. (1987). The clinical role of immunoscintigraphy in gastrointestinal cancer. *Monoclonal Antibodies in Immunoscintigraphy*. Edited by J.-F. Chatal, CRC Press, Boca Raton, FL.
16. Garnett, M. C., and Baldwin, R. W. (1986). An improved synthesis of a methotrexate-albumin-791T/36 monoclonal antibody conjugate cytotoxic to osteogenic sarcoma cell lines. *Cancer Res. 46*:2407–2412.
17. Roe, R., Robins, R. A., Laxton, R. R., and Baldwin, R. W. (1985). Kinetics of divalent monoclonal antibody binding to tumour cell surface antigens using flow cytometry: standardization and mathematical analysis. *Molec. Immunol. 22/1*:11–21.
18. Robins, R. A., Laxton, R. R., Garnett, M., Price, M. R., and Baldwin, R. W. (1986). Measurement of tumour reactive antibody and antibody conjugate by competition, quantitated by flow cytofluorimetry. *J. Immunol. Meth. 90*:165–172.
19. Embleton, M. J., Rowland, G. F., Simmonds, R. G., Jacobs, E., Marsden, C. H., and Baldwin, R. W. (1983). Selective cytotoxicity against human tumour cells by a vindesine-monoclonal antibody conjugate. *Br. J. Cancer 47*:43–49.
20. Pimm, M. V., Clegg, J. A., Caten, J. E., Ballantyne, K. D., Perkins, A. C., Garnett, M. C., and Baldwin, R. W. (1987). Biodistribution of methotrexate-monoclonal antibody conjugates and complexes: experimental and clinical studies. *Cancer Treatment Reviews 14*:411–420.
21. Aherne, G. W., Piall, E. M., and Marks, V. (1977). Development and application of a radioimmunoassay for methotrexate. *Br. J. Cancer 36*:608–617.
22. Pimm, M. V., Clegg, J. A., Garnett, M. C., and Baldwin, R. W. (1988). Biodistribution and tumour localisation of a methotrescate-monoclonal antibody 791T/36 conjugate in nude mice. *Int. J. Cancer 41*:886–891.

23. Ballantyne, K. C., Perkins, A. C., Pimm, M. V., Garnett, M. C., Armitage, N. C., Baldwin, R. W., and Hardcastle, J. D. (1986). Biodistribution and tumour localization of a monoclonal antibody-drug conjugate (791T/36-methotrexate). *Nucl. Med. Commun.* 7:310.
24. Byers, V. S., Pimm, M. V., Scannon, P. J., Pawluczyk, I., and Baldwin, R. W. (1987). Inhibition of growth of human tumour xenografts in athymic mice treated with ricin toxin A-chain-monoclonal antibody 791T/36 conjugates. *Cancer Res.* 47:5042–5046.
25. Willingham, M. C., Fitzgerald, D. J., and Pastan, I. (1987). *Pseudomonas* exotoxin coupled to a monoclonal antibody against ovarian cancer inhibits the growth of human ovarian cancer cells in a mouse model. *Proc. Natl. Acad. Sci. USA* 84:2474–2478.
26. Hara, H., and Seon, B. K. (1987). Complete suppression of *in vivo* growth of human leukemia cells by specific immunotoxins: nude mouse models. *Proc. Natl. Acad. Sci. USA* 84:3390–3394.
27. Thorpe, P. E., Detre, S. I., Foxwell, B. M. J., Brown, A. N. F., Skilleter, D. N., Wilson, G., Forrester, J. A., and Stirpe, F. (1985). Modification of the carbohydrate in ricin with metaperiodate-cyanoborohydride mixtures: effects on toxicity and in vivo distribution. *Eur. J. Biochem.* 147:197–206.
28. Skilleter, D. N., and Foxwell, B. M. J. (1986). Selective uptake of ricin A-chain by hepatic non-parenchymal cells in vitro. *FEBS* 196:344–348.
29. Byers, Vera S., Pimm, M. V., Pawluczyk, Izabella, Lee, H. M., Scannon, P. J., and Baldwin, R. W. (1987). Biodistribution of ricin toxin A chain-monoclonal antibody 791T/36 immunotoxin and the influence of hepatic blocking agents. *Cancer Res.* 47:5277–5283.
30. Bourrie, B. J. P., Casellas, P., Blythman, H. E., and Jansen, F. K. (1986). Study on the plasma clearance of antibody-ricin A chain immunotoxins. Evidence for specific recognition sites on the A chain that mediate rapid clearance of the immunotoxin. *Eur. J. Biochem.* 155:1–10.
31. Ponpipom, M. M., Bugianesi, R. L., Robbins, J. C., Doebber, T. W., and Shen, T. Y. (1981). Cell-specific ligands for selective drug delivery to tissues and organs. *J. Med. Chem.* 24:1399–1395.
32. Rowland, G. F., and Simmonds, R. G. (1986). Effects of monoclonal antibody-drug conjugates on human tumour cell cultures and xenografts. In *Monoclonal Antibodies for Cancer Detection and Therapy*. Edited by R. W. Baldwin and V. S. Byers. Academic Press, London, pp. 345–362.
33. Gallego, J., Price, M. R., and Baldwin, R. W. (1984). Preparation of four daunomycin-monoclonal antibody 791T/36 conjugates with anti-tumour activity. *Int. J. Cancer* 33:737–744.
34. Steinman, R. M., Mellman, I. S., Muller, W. A., and Cohn, Z. A. (1983). Endocytosis and the recycling of plasma membrane. *J. Cell Biol.* 96:1–27.
35. Goldstein, J. L., Anderson, R. G. W., and Brown, M. S. (1979). Coated pits, coated vesicles and receptor-mediated endocytosis. *Nature* 279:697–699.
36. Garnett, M. C., and Baldwin, R. W. (1986). Endocytosis of a monoclonal antibody recognising a cell surface glycoproteins antigen visualised using fluorescent conjugates. *Eur. J. Cell Biol.* 41:214–221.

37. Garnett, M. C., Embleton, M. J., Jacobs, E., and Baldwin, R. W. (1983).
    Preparation and properties of a drug-carrier-antibody conjugate showing
    selective antibody-directed cytotoxicity *in vitro*. *Int. J. Cancer 31*:661–670.
38. Garnett, M. C., Embleton, M. J., Jacobs, E., and Baldwin, R. W. (1985).
    Studies on the mechanism of action of an antibody-targeted drug-carrier
    conjugate. *Anti-Cancer Drug Des. 1*:3–12.
39. Jansen, F. K., Laurent, G., Liance, M. C., Blythman, H. E., Berthe, J.,
    Canat, X., Carayon, P., Carrier, D., Casellas, P., Derocq, J. M., Dussossoy,
    D., Fauser, A. A., Gorin, N. C., Gros, O., Gros, P., Laurent, J. C., Ponce-
    let, P., Remandet, B., Richer, G., and Vidal, H. (1986). Efficiency and toler-
    ance of the treatment with immuno-A-chain-toxins in human bone marrow
    transplantation. In *Monoclonal Antibodies for Cancer Detection and
    Therapy*. Edited by R. W. Baldwin and V. S. Byers. Academic Press,
    London, pp. 88–84.

4

Preclinical Studies with Immunoconjugates

GEOFFREY A. PIETERSZ, MARK J. SMYTH, JERRY KANELLOS,
ZITA CUNNINGHAM, and IAN F. C. McKENZIE
*Research Centre for Cancer and Transplantation, University of Melbourne,
Victoria, Australia*

I. INTRODUCTION

The concept of using antibodies to convey drugs to tumors was originally suggested by Paul Ehrlich in the early 1900s but, with only one or two exceptions, nothing has been done in this area until the last few years (1-4). There were some experiments performed by Alan Davies and colleagues using chlorambucil coupled noncovalently to goat antibodies produced against human tumors, with some in vitro and in vivo effects, but these studies appear not to have been pursued (3,4). The recent description of monoclonal antibodies with predominant and potent reaction against tumors (but usually not exclusive reactions against these cells) has led to the description of "vehicles" which could conceivably carry drugs/toxins/isotopes selectively to tumors and lead to their eradication (5,6). Thus the monoclonal antibodies may well hold the key to this old concept. However, it should be noted that virtually none of the monoclonal antibodies described thus far, particularly to solid tumors, are tumor specific and they do react with the normal tissue of origin and with other tissues (5). This has not led to any major clinical problems at this stage.

The other impetus for these studies is that there has been a general dissatis-
faction with the use of drugs for the treatment of a number of solid tumors—
particularly recurrences of carcinomas of the colon, breast, and melanoma. In
several of these cases there is virtually no treatment modality available. In this
setting it is reasonable to explore the value of using monoclonal antibodies
conjugated to drugs to enhance the specificity of the drugs. Finally, it is
widely recognized that most of the drugs currently used for therapeutic purposes
in cancer treatment today do have established side effects (7). Many oncologists
feel that the absence of side effects means that the drugs are doing little to
combat the cancer. There are clear indications for the use of drug/toxin/isotope-
antibody conjugate for the treatment of cancer in humans.

While the concept is now acceptable in principle and many trials are in
progress both at the preclinical and clinical stages, there are many problems to
be overcome before achieving the goal of curing cancer in humans with the use
of immunoconjugates (8,9). This review will address a number of these problems. First, monoclonal antibodies, particularly of murine origin, are not easy
to work with. Many are unstable, deteriorate on freezing and thawing, and are of
low affinity. However, by careful selection of the antibodies required, with
attention to specificity, stability, immunoglobulin class and affinity, it is possible to produce useful, if not ideal, monoclonal antibodies. The second problem is that of conjugating drugs to antibodies. The older methods of using
glutaraldehyde or carbodiimide, which tends to couple drug and antibody in
varying proportions to each other leading to polymerization, are really not
suitable for the routine and persistent production of good drug antibody conjugates, with retention of both drug and antibody activity. The problem is a major
one, mainly because most active drugs are hydrophobic compounds which have
to be attached to hydrophilic antibody moieties, and this requires the development of a number of new coupling procedures. In many cases there is great loss
of antibody, its activity, and of drug activity, after the coupling, and in very few
instances (see below) is there increased efficacy of the drug after coupling to
antibody. The third point worth mentioning is that although there may be loss
of drug activity with coupling, the drug which is coupled, at least in vitro, goes
to the tumor specifically via the antibody and the noncoupled drug reacts far
less specifically. The same findings occur in vivo (10). Thus, what is lost in activity may be more than gained by an increased specificity of the immunoconjugate. Having made a suitable drug–antibody conjugate the next problem is how
to get this into the tumor. At this time we regard this as being the *major* problem in the use of drug–antibody conjugates for the treatment of tumors (11).
Finally, tumors are heterogeneous with regard to their expression of antigen
with which the antibodies react (12). In any population of tumors some will
have large amounts of antigen, and therefore bind more of the antibody and

conjugate, and would be susceptible to destruction by the immunoconjugate. At the other end of the spectrum, many cells which lack the antigen altogether would not bind the immunoconjugate and therefore would not be affected at all.

If all of the above problems can be surmounted then the last problem concerns the reaction of the patient against the immunoconjugate (13). First, against the murine monoclonal antibody and second the drug-antibody conjugate could act as a hapten carrier system and antibodies made to the drugs themselves. Thus, there are a large number of problems, many of which have been overcome, which will be addressed in this review. At this time, a number of preclinical studies have been completed with several different drugs and clinical trials are currently in progress. It is not clear as yet whether immunoconjugates will lead to a cure for cancer or even a temporary reversal in the growth of tumors. However, the early results are promising and encourage us to proceed with full Phase I and II, even Phase III clinical studies. This review will address various aspects of our own work on the use of immunoconjugates, particularly using anthracycline analogs, folic acid antagonists, alkylating agents, and whole ricin. Studies using ricin A chain and conjugates with radioactive isotopes will be found elsewhere in this volume.

A. Models

We have used a number of different models, which roughly in toto are equivalent to in vivo use in patients. In model one, a murine thymoma, which originated after radiation, in B6.PL (75NS) mice was used (14). This tumor has the Ly-2^a (obtained from PL/J) and these mice are therefore Ly-2.1$^+$. By contrast, their congenic partner, C57BL/6 is Ly-2.2$^+$. This thymoma grows subcutaneously and in ascites form in C57BL/6 mice—the Ly-2.1 antigen does not act as a transplantation antigen and in C57BL/6 mice the tumor grows and will eventually kill the mice (15). This model in congenic mice provides one of the purest examples of a tumor-specific system, in that the tumor carries an antigen which is not carried at all by the host. As part of this model we have a series of Ly-2.1 monoclonal antibodies of different immunoglobulin classes, and thus in this model, variation of immunoglobulin class and affinity can also be examined. In a second model, we use cell lines growing in nude mice (mostly the HT29 and COLO 205 carcinoma of the colon cell line) (16). In a final model (studied in collaboration with Dr. Hamish Foster), fresh carcinoma of the colon samples are able to grow subcutaneously in nude mice. In addition, a number of other tumors are used both in vitro and in vivo as specificity controls and in most cases specificities are done in two ways: (a) using the one antibody and two different tumors, one reactive, the other not; and (b) using two antibodies (one reactive, the other not) and the one tumor.

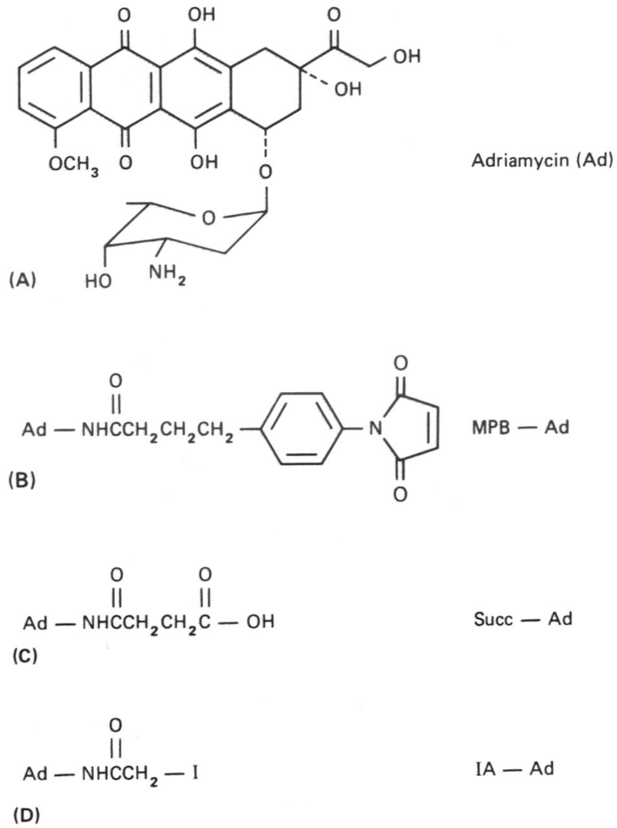

Figure 1 Chemical structures of adriamycin (A) and derivatives (B) maleimido-phenylbutyryl adriamycin (MPB-Ad), (C) succinyl adriamycin (Succ-Ad), (D) Iodacetyl adriamycin (IA-Ad).

II. RESULTS

A. Problems of Drug-Antibody Conjugation

A major problem in this reaction, as mentioned above, is the coupling of essentially hydrophobic components to water-soluble antibody molecules with the retention of both drug and antibody activity. Thus, in all of the coupling procedures antibody activity and recovery of protein should be monitored during the procedure and at its conclusion. We have found that in most coupling procedures there is a loss of up to 50% of the antibody activity, however, using monoclonal antibodies with such high titers one can obtain conjugates with the

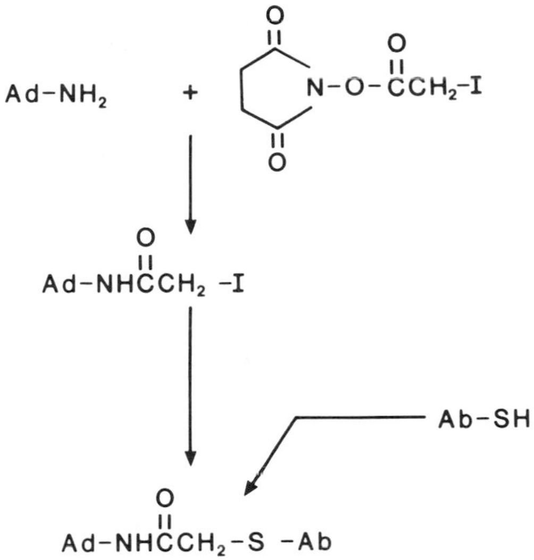

Figure 2 Preparation of iodoacetyl adriamycin and coupling to monoclonal antibody.

retention of useful antibody activity. The same principles hold for monitoring of drug–drug activity. In our studies we use inhibition of uptake of either [^{3}H] thymidine, uridine, or leucine uptake in appropriate studies. In our hands the inhibition of uptake of any of these moieties can be equated with toxicity to the tumors.

1. Most Drugs are Coupled to Antibody with Difficulty

Our initial attempts at coupling the anthracycline adriamycin to antibody failed completely. We used glutaraldehyde or carbodiimide following well-described protocols and were left with an insoluble red precipitate in the tube, which was devoid of any activity when a crude suspension was made with this material. Clearly, more specific methods of coupling were required.

2. Anthracycline Derivatives

To further couple adriamycin to antibody a number of analogs were produced, maleimidophenylbutyryl adriamycin (MPB-Ad), succinyl adriamycin (Succ-Ad), and iodoacetyl adriamycin (Fig. 1). For the first two analogs, satisfactory coupling procedures were designed and suitable amounts of drug were coupled to antibody (17). However, neither of these produced satisfactory drug activity. The

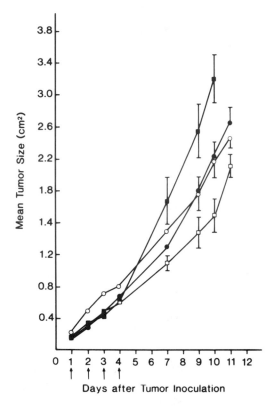

Figure 3 Growth of the murine thymoma ITT(1)75NS in (C57BL6 ×
BALB/c)F$_1$ mice injected s.c. with 3 × 10^6 cells. Groups of 10 mice were given
treatment i.p. denoted (↑); PBS (■), adriamycin (○), a mixture of adriamycin and
anti-Ly-2.1 (●), and IA-Ad-anti-Ly-2.1 conjugate (□). The total dose of adriamycin and anti-Ly-2.1 were 13 μg and 410 μg, respectively. Error bars represent
± standard error of the mean tumor size.

third compound, iodoacetyl adriamycin (IA-Ad), was coupled to antibody and
appeared suitable for further studies (Fig. 2). It was noted that in vitro the
inhibitory activity of IA-Ad was approximately 40-fold less than that of free
adriamycin; there was a major loss in drug activity on coupling to antibody.
Nonetheless there was specificity in this compound and the compound had some
activity in vivo in that approximately 30% of mice carrying the thymoma intraperitoneally had the tumor eradicated. Similarly, the conjugate was capable of
reducing the growth of established tumors (Fig. 3). However, the results were
not spectacular and we were concerned with the great loss of drug activity on
coupling. Clearly, if such conjugates were to be useful, we had to find better

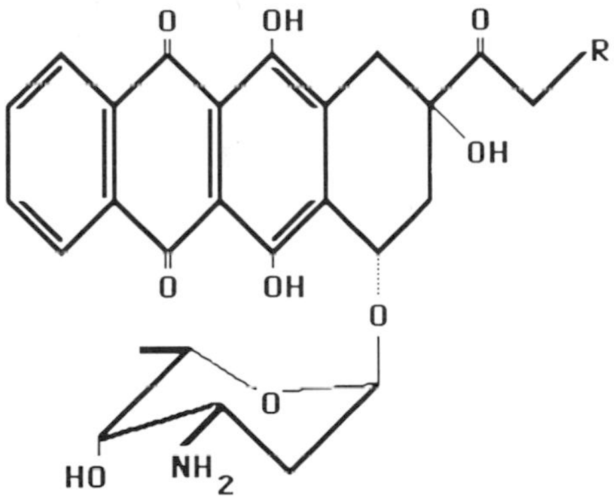

A   IDARUBICIN   R = H

B   BROMOIDARUBICIN   R = Br

C   AMINE LINK   R = NH-MoAb

D   ESTER LINK $R = O-\overset{\overset{O}{\|}}{C}-MoAb$

Figure 4 Structure of anthracycline derivatives (A) idarubicin, (B) bromo
idarubicin, and possible linkage to antibody (C and D)

methods of drug conjugation so that there was less loss of drug activity, or
alternatively use more toxic derivatives. Farmitalia kindly supplied bromoidarubicin, an analog of idarubicin, which satisfied both of these conditions.
Satisfactory coupling to antibody could be achieved via the C-14 to form an
ester link (Fig. 4). Two to five residues of idarubicin was coupled to antibody,
without a great loss of antibody activity and resulted in only a fourfold loss
in drug activity, compared to 40-fold with iodacetyl adriamycin. This conjugate was more toxic in vitro, and in vivo proved to be more effective in eradi-
cating tumors (18). When mice bearing established human colon carcinoma
xenografts received idarubicin antibody conjugate, tumors in 30% of the animals were eradicated, and most animals had a dramatic diminution in the size
of the tumors (Fig. 5). Thus, subcutaneous tumors could be cured by the use
of idarubicin antibody conjugates. Of importance in these studies was the finding that free idarubicin, used at the same dosage, had no effect on the growth
of the tumor which grew at the same rate as in untreated controls. However,
while the free idarubicin was without effect on the tumors it had a major effect

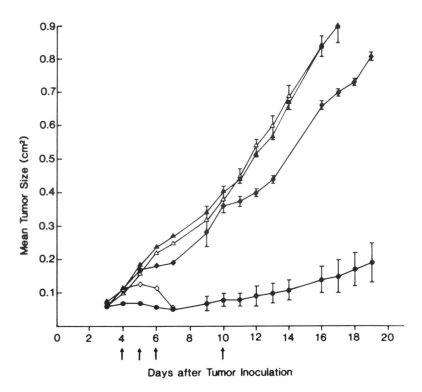

Figure 5 Growth of the human colon carcinoma xenograft COLO 205 in nude mice injected s.c. with 2×10^6 cells. Groups of 10 mice were given treatments denoted (↑); PBS (△), idarubicin (◆), Ida-250-30.6 conjugate (●), a mixture of Ida and 250-30.6 (◇) and 250-30.6 (▲). The total dose of idarubicin and 250-30.6 were 275 μg and 11.8 mg, respectively. Error bars represent ± standard error of the mean tumor size.

on the mice in that 80% of the mice receiving this therapy died from idarubicin toxicity. Thus, this experiment must be considered to be one of the most important in the developing history of the use of immunoconjugates. First, by careful selection of the drug for its toxicity and of the coupling procedure to maintain drug activity a useful conjugate could be obtained. Second, this conjugate was entirely specific in vivo and could eradicate tumors, in comparison with the unconjugated (free drug) which was toxic to almost all of the mice who received it. These results greatly encourage us to press on with this philosophy to search for more toxic materials which can be satisfactorily coupled to antibody. This also gives us confidence that the optimal drug-antibody conjugate which will cure some tumors can be found.

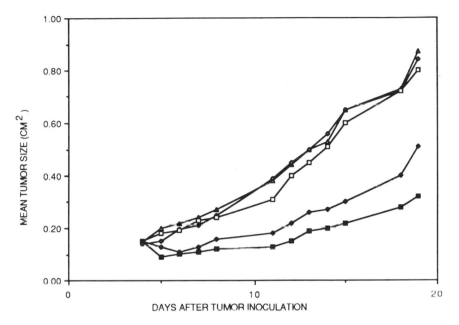

Figure 6 Growth of the COLO 205 human tumor xenograft in nude mice injected subcutaneously with 2×10^6 cells. Groups of 10 mice were given the following treatment i.v. on days, 4, 5, 8, 11, and 13; PBS ($\triangle$), methotrexate ($\diamondsuit$), aminopterin ($\square$), aminopterin-250-30.6 ($\blacksquare$), and methotrexate-250-30.6 ($\blacklozenge$). Standard error for each point was not more than ± 0.03 cm^3. Total doses of aminopterin and 250-30.6 were 37 μg and 1.9 mg, respectively, while the dose for methotrexate and conjugate was twice that of aminopterin.

3. Use of Folic Acid Antagonists

Folic acid antagonists, particularly methotrexate, are in current use for the treatment of cancer, although the more toxic derivative, aminopterin, has been abandoned in most clinical centers because of its toxicity. First, methotrexate was coupled to antibody using an active ester derivative. In this way 10 molecules of drug could be coupled per antibody molecule (16). Under these circumstances there was some loss of drug activity but a suitable drug–antibody conjugate was obtained. When tested in vitro, this was found to be a specific and toxic, yet on testing in vivo, although there was some shrinkage in the size of tumors grown subcutaneously none of the mice were cured. Thus, there was a reasonably potent conjugate produced which had a specific effect on but failed to eradicate any tumors. Clearly, more toxic derivatives were required, and in this light, aminopterin was examined. Using the same coupling procedure less aminopterin could be coupled to antibody (19). Nonetheless this was *more* effective than

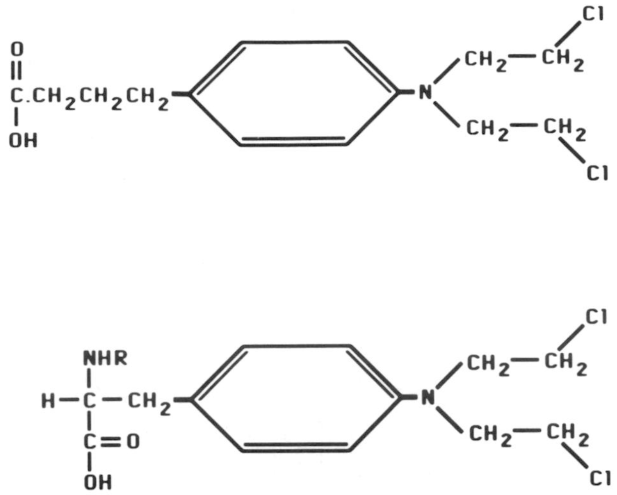

R = H   MELPHALAN
R = CH₃CO N-ACETYL MELPHALAN

Figure 7   Structure of melphalan and *N*-acetyl melphalan.

methotrexate antibody conjugates, both in vitro where aminopterin conjugates were 23 times more effective than methotrexate antibody conjugates, and in vivo (Fig. 6) there was a greater shrinkage of the tumors, and indeed, 10% of the animals were cured of their tumors. Thus, with the folic acid antagonists an important principle, elucidated above, was again proven: that more toxic derivatives give rise to greater effects.

4.   Use of Alkylating Agents

We have also coupled chlorambucil to monoclonal antibodies (15). Chlorambucil (Fig. 7) is unique in that for the first time we observed an increase in drug activity when coupled to monoclonal antibody (20). This was undoubtedly because large amounts of chlorambucil (up to 20–30 mol/mol of antibody) could be conjugated, and combined with the specificity of the antibody, gave rise to increased effects of the immunoconjugate over the free drug, this was apparent both in vitro and in vivo. Indeed, in vivo such conjugates could eradicate tumors growing in the ascites form in mice and caused a substantial reduction in the size of tumors growing subcutaneously. However, when the potency of conjugate was compared with others, such as methotrexate and idarubicin, it was clear that idarubicin was more effective. Thus, a less toxic drug such as chlorambucil, even when coupled in large amounts to antibody, may not be as effective as a more

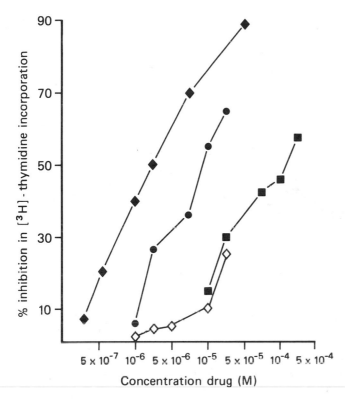

Figure 8 Inhibitory effect of melphalan (◆), N-acetyl melphalan (■), mixture of N-acetyl melphalan and antitransferrin receptor (◇) and N-acetyl melphalan-antitransferrin receptor conjugate (●) on CEM cells in the 24 h assay.

potent conjugate. Clearly, the ideal would be to have more molecules of a more toxic drug coupled to the antibody.

Thus, in this section we have demonstrated some of the difficulties and problems associated with the coupling of drugs to antibodies and have come up with several firm conclusions relating to the potency of the drug coupled, the number of molecules coupled and retention of drug and antibody activity after coupling. There were a variety of responses, from virtually no activity in vitro and in vivo, to the situation where tumors growing in the intraperitoneal site could be eradicated by several different treatments whereas those growing subcutaneously were more resistant. Clearly, more toxic compounds were required supplemented by more optimal coupling conditions.

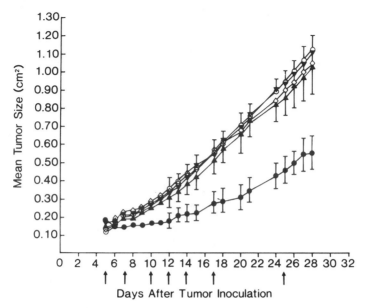

Figure 9 Growth of the COLO 205 human tumor xenograft in nude mice injected s.c. with 2 × 10⁶ cells. Groups of 10 mice were given treatments denoted
(↑); PBS (○), N-acetyl melphalan (▼), a mixture of N-acetyl melphalan and 250-
30.6 (◊), 250-30.6 (▲) and N-acetyl melphalan-250-30.6 conjugates (●). Total
doses of N-acetyl melphalan and antibody were 60 μg and 875 μg, respectively.
Error bars represent ± standard error of the mean.

B. Design of a Novel Immunoconjugate

The results obtained with chlorambucil encouraged us to examine a more toxic
alkylating agent, melphalan (21). Melphalan, also known as phenylalanine mus-
tard, enters cells by active transport using the amino acid transport system.
The potency of this agent resulted in the design of a novel drug, whereby an
acetyl group attached to the amino group of melphalan to form N-acetyl melphalan blocked the binding site of melphalan to cells (Fig. 7). However, when
coupled to antibody, N-acetyl-melphalan could enter cells via the antibody
route. This conjugate was highly specific in vitro (Fig. 8), and in vivo (Fig. 9)
could eradicate tumors growing in the peritoneum and reduce the size of those
growing subcutaneously and led to the cure of 30% of mice. This novel approach
may be of use with other compounds.

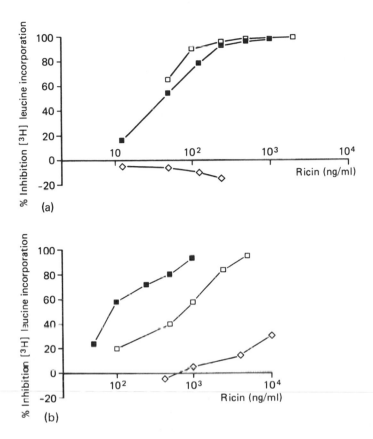

Figure 10 Inhibition of protein synthesis by ricin (□), ricin-anti-Ly-2.1 (■) and ricin-anti-Ly-1.1 (◇) in the absence (a) and presence (b) of lactose.

C. Use of Potent Whole Ricin Antibody Conjugates in Mice

Following from the above, we chose to produce whole ricin antibody conjugates. Ricin is one of the most toxic substances known; on a molar basis it is approximately 30,000 times more effective than such conventional drugs as adriamycin. We reasoned that if ricin could be satisfactorily coupled to antibody and used, its great toxicity would render highly active immunoconjugates. A new method was designed for coupling ricin to antibody using disulfide linkages formed with SAMSA and SPDP. Coupling was performed so that the galactose binding site for the ricin was blocked (22). In this way the ricin reacted specifically with target cells in vitro, whether lactose was present or

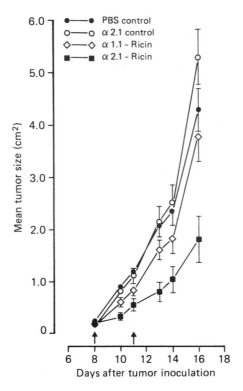

Figure 11   Growth of the murine thymoma ITT(1)75NS in (C57BL6 × BALB/c)F$_1$ mice injected s.c. with 6 × 10^6 cells. Groups of 10 mice were given treatments i.v. denoted (↑); PBS (●), anti-Ly-2.1 (○), ricin-anti-Ly-1.1 (◇) and ricin-anti-Ly-2.1 (■). Total doses of ricin and anti-Ly-2.1 were 0.1 μg and 0.44 μg, respectively. Error bars represent ± standard error of the mean tumor size.

absent, thus a potent conjugate which was shown to be effective with six different antibodies mixtures was obtained (Fig. 10). It is known that ricin A chain antibody conjugates are somewhat unreliable and in many systems the conjugates are ineffective or require a potentiating agent (23,24). How effective would these potent toxin-antibody conjugates be in vivo. First, using a lymphoma growing intraperitoneally, ricin-antibody conjugates caused the tumors to be eradicated and the mice cured of their tumors. However, when these conjugates were used intravenously, although up to 70% reduction in tumor size was observed (Fig. 11), none of the mice were cured of their tumors and some developed toxicity—probably due to ricin binding to liver receptors via mannose

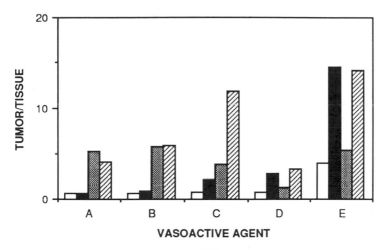

Figure 12 In vivo distribution of ^{125}I-anti-Ly-2.1 in tumor-bearing mice. ^{125}I-anti-Ly-2.1 was injected 1–4 h after the administration of vasoactive agent and mice were sacrificed after 24 h and the ^{125}I distribution obtained for all major organs. Tumor to tissue ratios for blood, in the presence (☐) or absence (■) of vasoactive agent and liver, in the presence (▨) or absence (▦) of vasoactive agent are shown. A, Prazosin; B, Cyclospasmol; C, Propranolol; D, Pindolol; E, Oxprenolol.

present on ricin. Thus, we could make two conclusions from this study. First, using the most toxic material available (ricin-antibody conjugates) the tumors can be eradicated if growing in the appropriate site. However, such cures could also be obtained with chlorambucil-antibody conjugates. Second, although the most potent material is available there is a problem in the material gaining access to tumors. Indeed, the smaller conjugates formed with idarubicin antibody were more potent than the highly toxic ricin-antibody conjugates—presumably as ricin immunoconjugates did not gain access to the tumors, either because of their size or because the ricin was diverted away from the tumor by carbohydrates. However, it is clear that access of immunoconjugate to the target is a *major* problem to be addressed in the next section.

D. The Problem of Access of Drugs to Tumor Cells

It was clear from the foregoing that even when the most toxic compounds known to humans (ricin immunoconjugates) are used intravenously with subcutaneous tumors, the conjugates still were unable to eradicate the tumors. In this particular case there may have been a problem with the size of the conjugate in that ricin-antibody conjugates have a molecular weight of approximately

220,000 (150,00 for IgG, 67,000 for ricin), as the smaller conjugates formed with idarubicin antibody were indeed more potent. In addition, ricin, a mannose-rich glycoprotein can bind to nonparenchymal cells in the liver even though the galactose binding sites on the B chain were blocked. However, it is very likely that in these experiments, size was an important factor in limiting access of the ricin-antibody conjugate to the target. When immunoconjugates are mixed with tumor cells under the most optimal circumstances, such as in a test tube, or when a tumor is growing in ascites, there can be complete eradication of the tumor as shown above for idarubicin, chlorambucil, and ricin-antibody conjugates. Therefore, a major obstacle to effecting a cure of solid tumors by drug-antibody conjugates is to obtain access for the immunoconjugates into the tumor.

On reflection it is not surprising that this presents a problem. There is no real reason why antibodies should bind to the tumors. There is no chemotactic effect and indeed if the circulation through a tumor is intact it would only be by accident that antibody does reach the tumor. Studies on determining the amount of antibody which does reach the tumor bear out this observation: in experimental animals up to 20% of antibody may reach the tumor, whereas in human this amount falls to less than .01% of the administered dose (25,26). How can this problem be overcome. In our first series of experiments we made use of vasoactive adrenergic agents for their paradoxical effect on tumors (27). Indeed, these agents are considered to have very little effect on tumor blood vessels but they do cause constriction or dilation of other vessels. In this way there is a greater blood volume *available* to the tumor when vasoconstrictors are used and tumor perfusion should increase. Biodistribution experiments indicated approximately threefold increase in tumor/blood and tumor/liver ratio when ^{125}I-labeled antibody was used with β-adrenergic agents (propanalol, pindalol, and oxprenolol). No change in biodistribution was seen with α-adrenergic agents (prazosin and cyclospasmol) (Fig. 12). We have found that the use of β-adrenergic agents (vasoconstriction agents) does increase tumor blood flow and has an increased effect when used with immunoconjugates (Fig. 13) (28). Thus, the next principle for the use of immunoconjugates is to increase the blood flow through the tumor and demonstrate that combined therapy is more suitable than single drug regimen.

In this light, we can report on experiments performed with tumor necrosis factor (TNF), wherein the combination of TNF and immunoconjugates has a synergistic effect and leads to eradication of a number of tumors (29). At this time we are perplexed as to the most optimal method of delivering specific therapy to tumors, and the use of TNF would appear to be the best manner of eliciting a local inflammatory response leading to vasodilation, increased permeability of vessels, and with this leakiness and increased blood flow, more drug-antibody conjugate would reach the tumor.

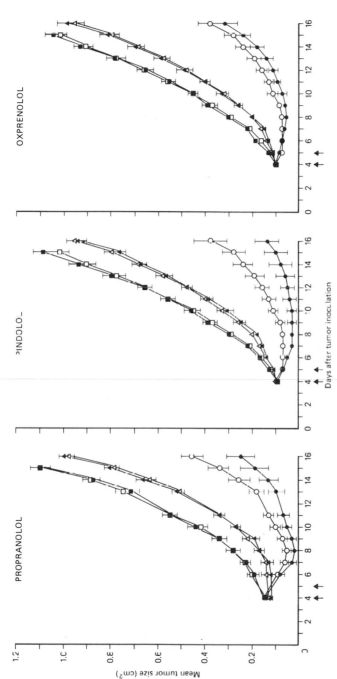

Figure 13 Growth of the thymoma ITT(1)75NS E3 in (C57BL6 × BALB/c)F$_1$ mice injected s.c. with 2×10^6 cells. Groups of 10 mice were given the following treatments i.v. denoted (↑); PBS (□), PBS and vasoactive agent (■), idarubicin (△), idarubicin and vasoactive agent (▲), idarubicin-anti-Ly-2.1 (○), and idarubicin-anti-Ly-2.1 and vasoactive agent (●). Error bars represent ± standard error of the mean tumor diameter. Total doses of idarubicin and antibody were 20 µg and 600 µg, respectively.

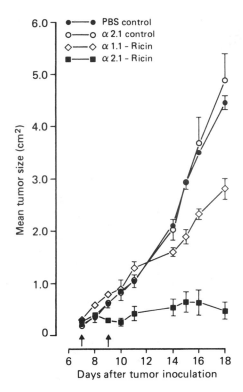

Figure 14 Growth of the murine thymoma ITT(1)75NS in (C57BL6 ×
BALB/c)F$_1$ mice injected s.c. with 6 × 10^6 cells. Groups of 10 mice were given
treatments intratumorally denoted (↑); PBS (●), ricin-anti-Ly-1.1 (◇), anti-
Ly-2.1 (○), and ricin-anti-Ly-2.1 (■). Total doses of ricin and antibody were
0.2 μg and 0.9 μg, respectively. Error bars represent ± standard error of the
mean tumor size.

E. Improving Access by Local Injection into Tumors

As indicated above, immunoconjugates given in the optimal site (such as in a
test tube or intraperitoneally) can eradicate tumors, whereas those given into
the circulation reach tumors only with difficulty. To perform a finite study
wherein our most toxic antibody-drug conjugates (the ricin-antibody conjugates
with the blocked galactose binding site) were used and delivered to subcutaneous
tumors directly into the tumors. Our philosophy here was that the ricin would
be delivered to the tumor and would be prevented from escaping by the antibody to tumor cells and entry into the cells also affected by the antibody–antigen interaction. We were able to demonstrate that whole ricin given into tumors

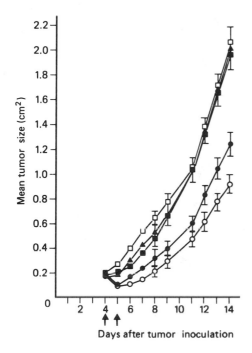

Figure 15 Growth of the tymoma ITT(1)75NS E3 in (C57BL6 X BALB/c)F$_1$ mice injected s.c. with 3 X 10^6 cells. Groups of 10 mice were given treatments i.v. denoted (↑); PBS (□), N-acetyl melphalan (■), N-acetyl melphalan-anti-Ly2.1 conjugate (●), N-acetyl melphalan-F(ab')$_2$ (○) and anti-Ly-2.1 F(ab')$_2$ (▲). Total doses of N-acetyl melphalan and antibody were 30 μg and 300 μg, respectively. Error bars represent + standard error of the mean.

had a marginal effect but had systemic toxicity due to escape from the tumor. By contrast, ricin antibody conjugates did not escape from tumors and were not toxic. Once the injection technique had been perfected by injecting in and around the tumor, the results of directly injecting tumors were dramatic— tumors disappeared within 48 hours to leave a shallow ulcer (Fig. 14). In a few cases these regrew and could be reinjected. Nonetheless local therapy (by intra-lesional injection) was able to eradicate tumors in a number of cases. This has several implications. First, with regard to immunoconjugates it is absolutely clear that if a potent immunoconjugate can be delivered to the site it can eradi-cate the tumor (22). Second, it is possible that ricin-antibody conjugates (or per-haps some other conjugates) combined with surgery and radiotherapy could serve as an alternative means of local therapy. In this light we are currently ex-

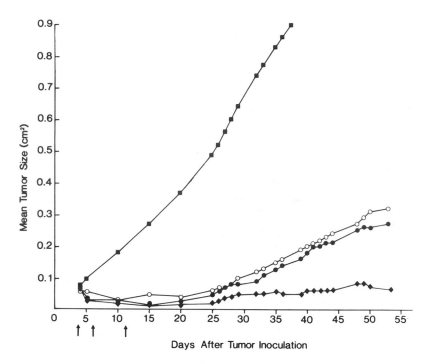

Figure 16 Tumor growth of COLO 205 human colon carcinoma xenograft in nude mice. Groups of 10 mice bearing pre-existing tumors were given one of the following treatments i.v. denoted (↑); PBS (■), idarubicin-250-30.6 conjugate (●), idarubicin-17.1 conjugate (○), and a mixture of idarubicin-17.1 conjugate and idarubicin-250-30.6 conjugate (♦). Total doses of idarubicin and antibody were 120 μg and 5.1 mg, respectively. Standard error for each point was not more than ± 0.03 cm^3.

amining the use of ricin-antibody conjugates as treatment for recurrent superficial tumors in breast cancer. Although long-term use of such conjugates would certainly not be advocated in breast cancer, the use of ricin-antibody conjugates in treating these superficial lesions in such patients would allow easy assessment of its actions. If this therapy proves useful, then palliative use of intralesional injection into tumors could be of value.

F. Does the Use of F(ab')$_2$ Fragments Improve Therapy with Immunoconjugates

If the large molecules, such as IgG drug-antibody complexes, cannot enter tumors easily, it is likely that smaller molecules such as F(ab')$_2$ drug-antibody complexes will have easier access. Indeed this is the reasoning behind the use of such complexes and in certain studies (30) such fragments have proven to be clinically more efficacious than whole antibody. In our hands the use of F(ab')$_2$ immunoconjugates has given equivocal results (Fig. 15), the effects of melphalan F(ab')$_2$ conjugates have been precisely the same as whole antibody (31). We are concerned with the philosophy behind the use of F(ab')$_2$ fragments. We firmly believe that whole antibody is likely to be more effective as it is a more natural product. We have argued that there is no reason why whole antibody, or fragments, should enter a tumor unless there is a major change in the vascular permeability. In our experiments, presumably the shorter half life of the antibody with F(ab')$_2$ immunoconjugates was balanced by the more ready entry into tumor cells. At this time it is not clear whether F(ab')$_2$ fragments have a future role in immunotherapy.

G. The Problem of Tumor Heterogeneity

If we can assume that the problems of coupling drugs and toxins to antibody can be overcome and a method can be found whereby a considerable proportion of the antibody does reach the tumor, there is still the major problem of tumor heterogeneity. Some tumors may simply not bind any antibody, or sufficient antibody, to have a toxic effect and these grow on in a modified fashion. We are firm believers that the solution to this would be to use "cocktails" of antibodies against as many antigens on the cell surface as one has antibodies. In a simple yet important experiment it is clearly demonstrated that the same dose of drug delivered on *two* separate antibodies against two different antigens is much more potent than the same dose delivered via a single antibody (Fig. 16). The message is: "cocktails" of antibodies are important. In this light, it would appear, at least theoretically, that isotopes will have a major role in this form of therapy wherein adjacent cells, perhaps so undifferentiated as to carry no antigens as represented by antibodies in the cocktail, can still be bombarded and killed (32,33).

III. CONCLUSIONS

We have reviewed our own work in this field, and given that this is a review we can pontificate and elaborate several principles for the use of immunoconjugates.

1. Drugs and antibodies must be conjugated so as to obtain maximum drug and antibody activity.
2. More toxic analogs are more potent than less toxic analogs. The search for more toxic drugs should be continued and, indeed, our feeling is that the drugs in common use today (chosen for their therapeutic index) should be

abandoned and the drugs from the shelves of the pharmaceutical compan-
ies should be used for these particular studies. Their heightened toxicity
and increased specificity on conjugates to monoclonal antibodies is
needed.

3. There is a major problem with access to solid tumors and any attempts to
improve access would yield improved results.

4. Drug-antibody conjugates delivered to the site of a tumor can lead to its
eradication. At this time intraperitoneally grown tumors (selected models)
and intralesional therapy can lead to the eradication of tumors. Many solid
tumors remain resistant.

5. "Cocktails" containing multiple antibodies will be more useful than single
antibody therapy.

6. It is most likely that combined therapy with many moieties will be useful
for an attack on context. In the broad context this will be a combination
of surgery, possibly radiotherapy, conventional drugs, immunoconjugates,
vasodilating agents, and possibly tumor necrosis factor. Given the rate of
progress in this field, we are confident that many of these problems will be
solved within the next few years. However, as Phase I and II studies are
now in progress it is pertinent to mention several practical issues. First, the
knowledge of Immunologists must be extended to include stability studies
on the products both in vitro and in vivo, and therefore it is crucial that
radiolabeled drugs are available. We have gone beyond immunology and a
new science of immunopharmacology is now upon us. Second, the current
therapeutic measures are expensive and at some stage the cost of the procedures will have to be measured against the benefits. In the early stages,
there are now sufficient data accrued from preclinical studies to enable an
optimistic outlook—tumors are being eradicated in experimental animals—
hopefully this will occur in humans.

REFERENCES

1. Ehrlich, P. (1906). *Collected Studies on Immunity*, Vol. 11. John Wiley, New York.
2. Mathé, G., Loc, T. B., and Bernard, J. (1958). Effet sur la Leucémie 1210 de la souris d'une combinaison par diazotation d'A-methopterine et de α-globu-lins de hamsters porteurs de cette leucémie par hélérogrette. *C.R. Acad. Sci. Paris 246*:1626-1628.
3. Davies, D. A. L., and O'Neill, G. J. (1973). *In vivo* and *in vitro* effects of tu-mor specific antibodies with chlorambucil. *Br. J. Cancer 28*:285-298.
4. Newman, C. E., Ford, C. H. J., Davies, D. A. L., and O'Neill, G. J. (1977). Antibody-drug synergism: an assessment of specific passive immunotherapy in bronchial carcinoma. *Lancet 2*:163-167.

5. Teh, J. G., Stacker, S. A., Thompson, C. H., and McKenzie, I. F. C. (1985). The diagnosis of human tumors with monoclonal antibodies. *Cancer Surveys* 4:149–184.
6. Pietersz, G. A., Kanellos, J., Smyth, M. J., Zalcberg, J., and McKenzie, I. F. C. (1987). The use of monoclonal antibody conjugates for the diagnosis and treatment of cancer. *Immunol. Cell Biol. 65(2)*:111–125.
7. Devita, V., Jr., Hellman, S., and Rosenberg, S. A. (1984). In *Cancer Principles and Practice*. J. B. Lippincott, Philadelphia.
8. Timms, R. M. (1987). Methotrexate immunoconjugate in lung cancer. Communication at Second International Conference on Monoclonal Antibody Immunoconjugates for Cancer, San Diego.
9. Baldwin, R. W., and Byers, V. S. (1987). Monoclonal antibody 791T/36 immunoconjugates for treatment of colorectal and ovarian cancer. Communication at International Conference on Covalently Modified Antigens and Antibodies in Diagnosis and Therapy, Lyon.
10. Deguchi, T., Chu, T. M., Leong, S. S., Horoszewicz, J. S., and Lee, C. (1986). Effect of methotrexate-monoclonal anti-prostatic acid phosphatase antibody conjugate on human prostate cancer. *Cancer Res. 46*:3751–3755.
11. Poznansky, M. J., and Juliano, R. L. (1984). Biological approaches to the controlled delivery of drugs. A critical review. *Pharmacol. Rev. 36*:277–336.
12. Durrant, L. G., Robins, R. A., Armitage, N. C., Brown, A., Baldwin, R. W., and Hardcastle, J. D. (1986). Association of antigen expression and DNA ploidy in human colorectal tumors. *Cancer Res. 46*:3543–3549.
13. Courlenay-Luck, N. S., Epenetos, A. A., Moore, R., Larche, M., Pectasides, D., Dhokia, B., and Ritter, M. A. (1986). Development of primary and secondary immune responses to mouse monoclonal antibodies used in the diagnosis and therapy of malignant neoplasms. *Cancer Res. 46*:6489–6493.
14. Hogarth, P. M., Henning, M. M., and McKenzie, I. F. C. (1982). Alloantigenic phenotype of radiation-induced thymomas in the mouse. *J. Natl. Cancer Inst. 69*:619–626.
15. Smyth, M. J., Pietersz, G. A., Classon, B. J., and McKenzie, I. F. C. (1986). Specific targeting of chlorambucil to tumors with the use of monoclonal antibodies. *J. Natl. Cancer Inst. 76*:503–510.
16. Kanellos, J., Pietersz, G. A., and McKenzie, I. F. C. (1985). Studies of methotrexate-monoclonal antibody conjugates for immunotherapy. *J. Natl. Cancer Inst. 75*:319–332.
17. Pietersz, G. A., Smyth, M. J., and McKenzie, I. F. C. (1987). The use of anthracycline antibody complexes for specific anti-tumor therapy. In *Targeting Diagnosis and Therapy*. Edited by J. D. Rodwell. Marcel Dekker, New York, Vol. 1.
18. Pietersz, G. A., Smyth, M. J., and McKenzie, I. F. C. (1988). Immunochemotherapy of a murine thymoma with the use of Idarubicin-monoclonal antibody conjugates. *Cancer Res. 48*:926–931.
19. Kanellos, J., Pietersz, G. A., Cunningham, Z., and McKenzie, I. F. C. (1987). Anti-tumour activity of aminopterin-monoclonal antibody conjugates, *in*

vitro and *in vivo* comparison with methotrexate-monoclonal antibody conjugates. *Immunol. Cell Biol.* 65(6):483–493.

20. Smyth, M. J., Pietersz, G. A., and McKenzie, I. F. C. (1986). Potentiation of *in vitro* cytotoxicity of chlorambucil with monoclonal antibodies. *J. Immunol.* 37:3361–3366.

21. Smyth, M. J., Pietersz, G. A., and McKenzie, I. F. C. (1987). Selective enhancement of anti-tumor activity of N-acetyl melphalan upon conjugation to monoclonal antibodies. *Cancer Res.* 47:62–69.

22. Pietersz, G. A., Kanellos, J., and McKenzie, I. F. C. (1986). The use of whole ricin-antibody conjugates for the treatment of tumors in mice. In *Membrane Mediated Cytotoxicity*. UCLA Symposia on Molecular and Cellular Biology, New Series, Allan R. Liss, New York, Vol. 45.

23. Casellas, P., Bourrie, B. J. P., Gros, P., and Jansen, F. K. (1984). Kinetics of cytotoxicity induced by immunotoxins. Enhancement by lysomotropic amines and carboxylic ionophores. *J. Biol. Chem.* 259:9359–9364.

24. Vitetta, E. S., Fulton, R. J., and Uhr, J. W. (1984). Cytotoxicity of a cell-reactive immunotoxin containing ricin A-chain is potentiated by an anti-immunotoxin containing ricin B chain. *J. Exp. Med.* 160:341–346.

25. Andrew, S. M., Pimm, M. V., Perkins, A. C., and Baldwin, R. W. (1986). Comparative imaging and biodistribution studies wiht an anti-CEA monoclonal antibody and its F(ab')$_2$ and Fab fragments in mice with colon carcinoma xenografts. *Eur. J. Nucl. Med.* 12:168–175.

26. Epenetos, A. A., Snook, D., Durbin, H., Johnson, P. M., and Taylor-Papadimitriou, J. (1986). Limitations of radiolabelled monoclonal antibodies for localization of human neoplasms. *Cancer Res.* 46:3183–3191.

27. Chan, R. C., Babbs, C. F., Vetter, R. J., and Lamar, C. H. (1984). Abnormal response of tumor vasculature to vasoactive drugs. *J. Natl. Cancer Inst. 72*: 145–150.

28. Smyth, M. J., Pietersz, G. A., and McKenzie, I. F. C. (1987). The use of vasoactive agents to increase tumor perfusion and the antitumor efficacy of drug-monoclonal antibody conjugates. *J. Natl. Cancer Inst.* 79:1367–1373.

29. Smyth, M. J., Pietersz, G. A., and McKenzie, I. F. C. (1988). The increased anti-tumor effect of immunoconjugates and tumor necrosis factor *in vivo*. *Cancer Res.* 48:3607–3612.

30. Mach, J-P., Chatal, J-F., Lumbroso, J-D., Buchegger, F., Forni, M., Ritschard, J., Berche, C., Douillard, J-Y., Carrel, S., Herlyn, M., Steplewski, Z., and Koprowski, H. (1983). Tumor localization in patients by radiolabeled monoclonal antibodies against colon carcinoma. *Cancer Res.* 43:5593–5600.

31. Smyth, M. J., Pietersz, G. A., and McKenzie, I. F. C. (1987). The *in vitro* and *in vivo* anti-tumour activity of N-AcMEL-F(ab')$_2$ conjugates. *Br. J. Cancer* 55:7–11.

32. Anderson-Berg, W. T., Squire, R. A., and Strand, M. (1987). Specific radioimmunotherapy using ^{90}Yt-labelled monoclonal antibody in erythroleukaemic mice. *Cancer Res.* 47:1905–1912.

33. Kozak, R. W., Atcher, R. W., Ganson, O. A., Friedman, A. M., Hines, J. J., and Waldman, T. A. (1986). Bismuth-212-labelled anti-tac monoclonal antibody: α-particle-emitting radionuclides as modalities for radioimmunotherapy. *Proc. Natl. Acad. Sci. USA 83*:474–487.

5

Radioimmunoscintigraphy and Radioimmunotherapy in Nude Mouse Models
Studies with Site-Specifically Modified Monoclonal Antibodies

VERNON L. ALVAREZ, A. DWIGHT LOPES, JOHN D. RODWELL,
AND THOMAS J. McKEARN
CYTOGEN Corporation, Princeton, New Jersey

FRANK P. STUART
University of Chicago, Chicago, Illinois

I. INTRODUCTION

Since the advent of monoclonal antibody technology (1), numerous diagnostic and therapeutic applications in the field of oncology have been proposed. These applications typically require coupling of the antibody to another substance— most notably imaging and therapeutic agents. To maximize clinical utility, any covalent modification of the antibody should not disrupt its immunoreactivity. Many of the processes described for monoclonal antibodies involve modification of a certain class of sites on the antibody. For example, coupling of toxins, isotopes, or cytotoxic drugs to antibodies has been achieved by direct covalent attachment to tyrosines, lysines, and carboxyl side chains of aspartic and glutamic acids (2-6). These residues are distributed throughout the antibody; therefore, some of the attachment sites could likely be located near or at the antigen-binding region (see Fig. 1). The result would be weakened or lost antigen-binding activity for a proportion of the antibody conjugates.

An alternative approach is site-specific covalent modification of monoclonal antibodies. Such site specificity can be accomplished by attachment at the

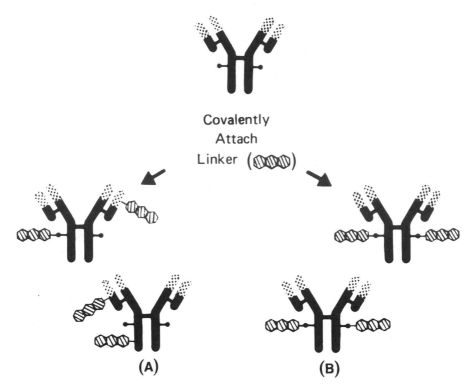

Figure 1 Attachment sites on monoclonal antibodies. (A) Direct covalent attachment to tyrosine, lysine or glutamic/aspartic acid residues. (B) Site-specific attachment to oligosaccharide moiety.

oligosaccharide moiety of the antibody molecule. This complex carbohydrate is localized on the heavy chains of the immunoglobulin at sites distal to the antigen-binding region (Fig. 1). By using these oligosaccharide sites, both the homogeneous antigen-binding properties and the affinity of the unmodified protein should be retained. In contrast, conjugates of antibodies prepared by direct coupling to tyrosine, lysine, or aspartic/glutamic acid residues would have heterogeneous antigen-binding properties and reduced affinity.

This chapter focuses on the advantages and properties of site-specific modification of monoclonal antibodies and will present data to support our view that, of the modification techniques developed thus far, this is the best suited for diagnostic and therapeutic applications. We will review previously published data from our laboratory on the use of 111-indium-labeled antibodies for radioimmunoscintigraphy and will present preliminary data using 212-bismuth- and 90-yttrium-labeled antibodies for radioimmunotherapy.

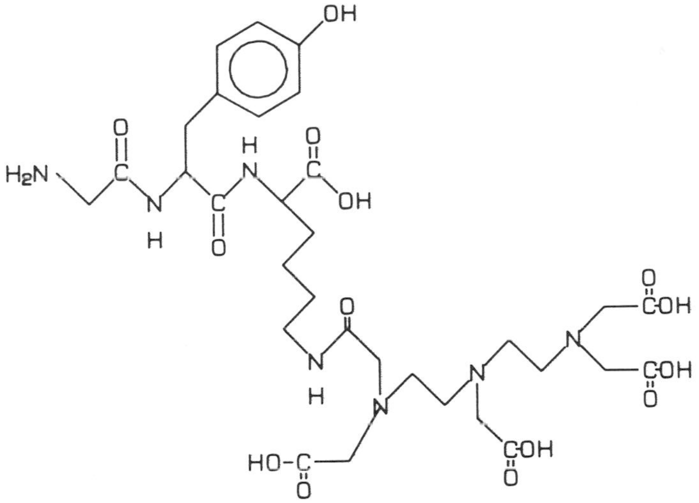

Figure 2 Structural formula for tripeptide chelator, glycyl-tyrosyl-(N-ϵ-diethyl-enepentaacetic acid)-lysine, GYK-DTPA.

II. SITE-SPECIFIC MODIFICATION OF MONOCLONAL ANTIBODIES

A. Brief Review of the Preparation of Site-Specific Modified Antibodies

To modify a monoclonal antibody at the oligosaccharide moiety, it is necessary first to oxidize the carbohydrate to aldehyde residues. These resultant aldehydes react with many different compounds, including amines, hydrazines, and hydrazides. In all of the studies discussed in this chapter, the monoclonal antibodies were modified with the chelator abbreviated GYK-DTPA (Fig. 2). GYK is the tripeptide glycyl-tyrosyl-lysine. DTPA is the chelator diethylenetriaminepenta-acetic acid. DTPA is attached to the ϵ-amino group of the lysine residue while the amino terminal glycyl residue attaches to the reactive aldehydes on the antibody. A complete description of the preparation of GYK-DTPA antibody conjugates can be found elsewhere (7). Briefly, this process involves three steps: oxidation of the antibody; overnight incubation of the antibody with a 2000-fold molar excess of GYK-DTPA; and purification of the antibody using Sephadex G-50, Superose 12 or another gel filtration method. A major advantage of this technique is that it is suitable for most types of antibodies. We have successfully coupled GYK-DTPA to more than 100 different monoclonal antibodies using the same protocol described above.

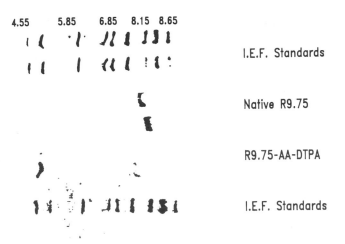

Figure 3 Isoelectric focusing gel (IEF) fluorographs for native and site-specific modified R9.75 monoclonal antibody.

B. Homogeneity of Oligosaccharide-Linked Conjugates

The homogeneity of the site-specific modified conjugates had previously been assessed for an IgM antibody using a Sipps analysis (8). To further evaluate the homogeneity, isoelectric focusing (IEF) gels of native and conjugated R9.75, a rat IgG2c monoclonal antibody, were performed. Figure 3 shows the IEF pattern obtained with this analysis. As seen in this figure, the native antibody focused at a pH of about 8.3. When modified site-specifically using the chelator amino aniline DTPA, the conjugated antibody shifted to an acidic pH of about 4.5. It is obvious that virtually all of the band moved to this new pH, which indicates that the conjugate is homogeneous. IEF data, which are reproducible with many antibodies, provide one means to measure the homogeneity of conjugation.

C. Extent of Derivatization of Antibody

The extent of derivatization of the antibody with GYK-DTPA can be evaluated using two methods. The first method involves direct iodination of the tyrosine residue on the GYK-DTPA to a known specific activity. The trace-labeled GYK-DTPA is then coupled with the oxidized antibody using the technique described in Section II.A. After the antibody is purified from unreacted GYK-DTPA, the number of GYK-DTPA molecules per antibody can be determined by the specific activity.

Using the second method, the antibody is first coupled with GYK-DTPA and the number of GYK-DTPA molecules quantitated by metal binding. In our

Table 1 Determination of the Number of GYK-DTPA Groups Per Antibody

Antibody	Subclass	Moles GYK-DTPA per mole antibody
R9.75	IgG2c	5.3
3454	IgG1	2.7
B72.3	IgG1	5.8
S4	IgG2a	7.1

laboratory we use cold indium that has been trace labeled with ^{111}In so that the specific activity is known. After the antibody has been labeled, the number of indium atoms and the ratio of indium atoms per antibody are determined. By inference, the number of GYK-DTPAs per antibody can be calculated. Both methods yield the same results provided that any trace metal contaminants present in the various solutions and buffers used in the second method have been removed.

Table 1 shows the extent of derivatization for four different antibodies; comparable techniques were used to measure the extent of derivatization for each. R9.75 is an IgG2c rat monoclonal antibody, 3454 is a mouse IgG1 antibody, B72.3 is an anticolorectal carcinoma IgG1 antibody and S4 is an antirenal cell carcinoma IgG2a antibody. The derivatization ratios were 3 to 7 GYK-DTPA molecules per antibody. We have been able to achieve derivatization ratios in this range for most of the antibodies we have evaluated. In one instance, we were able to attach 22.4 GYK-DTPA molecules per antibody using human serum albumin (HSA) as a site-specific linker to the R9.75 antibody. These derivatization ratios are much higher than the one or less than one ratios commonly reported for DTPA (9,10).

D. Immunoreactivity of GYK-DTPA Antibody Conjugates

A substantial loss of immunoreactivity has been reported when the derivatization ratio has exceeded one DTPA molecule per antibody (9,10). Site-specific modification at the oligosaccharide permits much higher loading with little or no loss of immunoreactivity. The immunoreactivity of the antibody conjugate can be assessed using several techniques. One such technique is a competitive binding assay in which iodine-labeled antibodies and derivatized antibodies compete for binding sites on the live target cells. Another technique is an ELISA-type assay. In this assay, target cells are fixed on a 96-well plate and binding of the native antibody is compared to that of the site-specific modified antibody

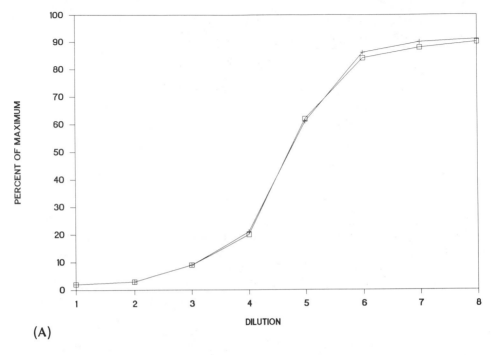

(A)

Figure 4 Immunoreactivity of native versus site-specific modified monoclonal antibodies. (A) Competition assay using ^{125}I-labeled R9.75 and either native R9.75 (□) or site-specific modified R9.75-HSA-DTPA (+) to complete binding. (B) ELISA assay using LS174T fixed-cell 96-well plates to compare reactivity of native B72.3 (□) or site-specific modified B72.3-GYK-DTPA (+). (C) ELISA assay using 7860 fixed-cell 96-well plates to compare reactivity of native S4 (□) or site-specific modified (+) S4-GYK-DTPA. OD is optical density at 495 nm.

conjugate. Figure 4 illustrates the results of three different assays using either the ELISA or the competitive binding assays. In each, the native antibody was compared with the GYK-DTPA conjugate. In all three, there was no apparent loss of immunoreactivity following site-specific modification of the antibody.

Yet a third technique for assessing the extent of immunoreactivity is a classical direct binding assay using ^{111}In-labeled GYK-DTPA antibody conjugate. Although the direct binding assay can measure the immunoreactivity of the labeled conjugate, it is not possible to directly compare the reactivity of the native and derivatized antibody using this assay. One advantage of the direct binding assay, however, is that it is sufficiently sensitive to detect small changes in immunoreactivity. The ELISA-type assay, by contrast, is suitable only for meas-

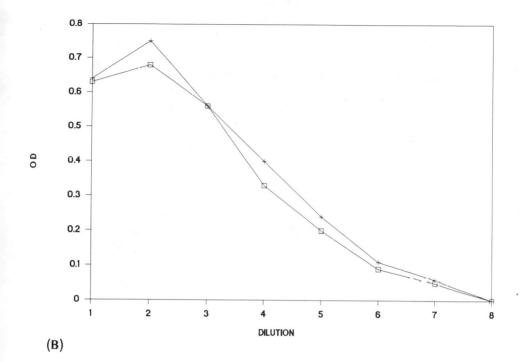

(B)

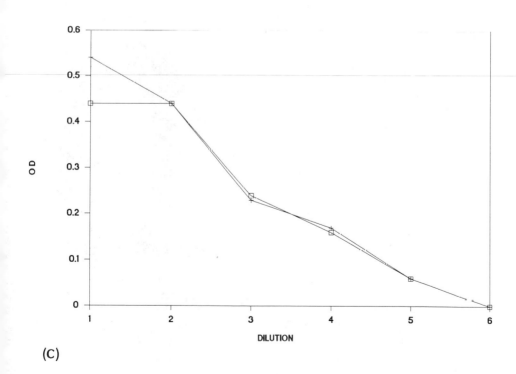

(C)

105

uring the immunoreactivity of bulk conjugate. Because only a small fraction of the conjugates are actually labeled with the isotope, the issue of sensitivity becomes critical in detecting the immunoreactivity of the labeled fraction. Using a direct binding assay, we have demonstrated that it is possible to bind approximately 80% of the counts for $[^{111}In]$ S4-GYK-DTPA conjugates to target cells (7).

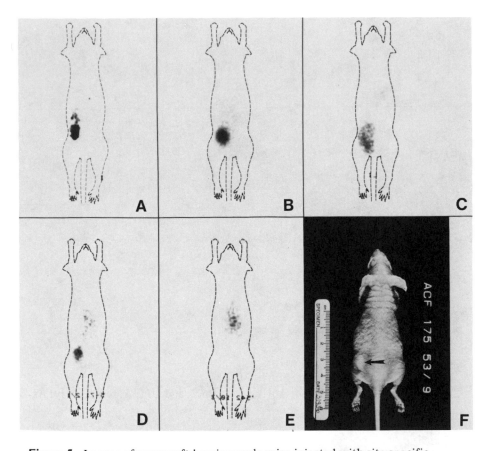

Figure 5 Images of xenograft-bearing nude mice injected with site-specific modified ^{111}In-labeled monoclonal antibodies: (A) antibody A6H, xenograft 7860 (renal cell carcinoma); (B) antibody B6.2, xenograft MCF7 (breast carcinoma); (C) antibody B72.3, xenograft LS174T (colon carcinoma); (D) antibody S4, xenograft SKRC-1 (renal cell carcinoma); (E) normal, non-xenograft-bearing nude mouse; (F) photograph of mouse showing typical size of tumor (arrow).

Table 2 Summary of Biodistribution Results from 111-Indium-Labeled Antibody Conjugates in Nude Mice Xenograft Models

Tumor type	Cell line	Monoclonal antibody	Tumor-to-blood ratio	Liver-to-blood ratio[a]
Renal cell	7860	A6H (N=6)	194:1	3.6:1
carcinoma	7860	S4 (N=12)	58:1	2.5:1
	SKRC-1	S4 (N=12)	52:1	3.2:1
	SKRC-45	S4 (N=6)	6:1	3.2:1
Breast/colon	LS174T	B72.3 (N=20)	4:1	2.3:1
carcinoma	ZR75.1	B6.2 (N=10)	5:1	0.7:1
Neuroblastoma	IMR5	UJ13A (N=4)	3:1	0.7:1

[a]Liver-to-blood ratios in control animals ranged from 0.6:1 to 1.7:1.

III. RADIOIMMUNOSCINTIGRAPHIC STUDIES WITH 111-INDIUM IN NUDE MOUSE MODELS

Having adequately demonstrated that site-specific modification not only increases the extent of derivatization possible without disrupting the immunoreactivity of the antibodies, we next demonstrated that the modified antibodies have diagnostic potential. We conducted a series of imaging and biodistribution studies with ^{111}In-labeled GTK-DTPA antibody conjugates using human tumor xenografts in nude mice.

A. Imaging and Biodistribution Studies in Tumor Xenograft Models

Nude mice injected with human tumor cells develop tumors at the site of implantation. Figure 5 shows images of mice which had been injected with different cell lines: SKRC (renal cell carcinoma), 7860 (renal cell carcinoma), MCF7 (breast carcinoma), and IMR5 (neuroblastoma). The site-specific modified[111] In-labeled antibodies used were S4, A6H, B72.3, B6.2, and UJ13A, respectively. As seen in these images, each of the antibodies localized to the tumor xenograft.

Another very interesting observation from the images shown in Figure 5 is that there was very little uptake of the radiolabeled antibodies by the liver. Many groups have reported only limited success using ^{111}In-labeled antibodies for radioimmunoscintigraphy, primarily due to nonspecific localization of the antibodies in the liver (e.g., Refs. 11–13). Table 2 shows the biodistribution data from our imaging studies. Both the tumor-to-blood and liver-to-blood ratios for each cell line and antibody type are shown in this table. A ratio greater than one indicates specific uptake by the tissue or organ. A ratio less than or equal to one

Table 3   Tissue-to-Blood Ratios in Nontumor-Bearing Mice (Mean ± Standard Deviation)

Tissue	Antibody			
	Human IgG (N = 3)	A6H (N = 6)	CYT029 (N = 3)	HT29.15 (N = 5)
Lung	0.5 ± 0.1	0.4 ± 0.1	0.6 ± 0.1	0.4 ± 0.1
Spleen	0.8 ± 0.1	0.3 ± 0.1	0.9 ± 0.3	0.3 ± 0.1
Liver	1.2 ± 0.2	0.5 ± 0.1	1.0 ± 0.2	0.4 ± 0.1
Kidney[a]	1.4 ± 0.2	0.3 ± 0.1	1.4 ± 0.2	0.3 ± 0.1
Muscle	0.1 ± 0.1	0.1 ± 0.1	0.1 ± 0.1	0.1 ± 0.1
Lymph node[b]	0.3 ± 0.1	0.3 ± 0.1	0.4 ± 0.2	0.3 ± 0.01

[a]Average of right and left kidney.
[b]Average of right and left axillary and inguinal lymph nodes.
Source: Ref. 14.

indicates that the counts in the tissue or organ are the result of antibodies present in the blood supply to that region. In each xenograft model, the tumor-to-blood ratio was greater than the liver-to-blood ratio, suggesting that specific localization of the labeled antibody to the tumor site had occurred.

B. Imaging and Biodistribution Studies in Normal Nude Mice

To determine whether the relative absence of nonspecific liver uptake found in our imaging studies was a general benefit of site-specific modification of the antibody, we conducted a series of in vivo antibody localization studies in normal nude mice. Since no tumor was present in these animals, the role of nonspecific localization due to factors unrelated to the specificity of the antibodies could be evaluated.

Nontumor-bearing nude mice were injected with one of four different antibodies, all of which had been labeled with ^{111}In and modified at the oligosaccharide using the procedure described in Section II.A (14). The antibodies were: a human myeloma IgG, an antirenal cell carcinoma IgG1 (A6H), an anti-T-cell IgG (Cyt029), and an anticolorectal carcinoma IgG1 (HT29.15). There was no selective uptake into the regions of the spleen or liver obvious in the images taken from these normal nude mice. The biodistribution data from these studies also support a lack of uptake by the liver or spleen (see Table 3). The tissue-to-blood ratios reflected the relative blood flow to the various tissues. Thus, site-

Table 4 Tissue-to-Blood Ratios 24 Hours After Antibody Injection in Nontumor-Bearing Mice and Mice Inoculated with BN Lymphoma Cells

Tissue	Direct label		Oligosaccharide label	
	Tumor xenograft	Control	Tumor xenograft	Control
Tumor	1	—	5.5	—
Liver	0.2	0.2	2.4	0.5
Lung	0.8	0.5	1.1	0.6
Spleen	0.3	0.3	1.9	0.4
Kidney	0.4	0.1	1.5	0.5
Blood	1	1	1	1

Source: Ref. 8.

specific modification of the monoclonal antibody does not appear to cause substantial localization of the antibody in nontarget tissues.

We next compared localization of iodinated monoclonal antibody conjugates prepared either by site-specific modification at the oligosaccharide or by directly iodinating the antibody at tyrosine using the chloramine-T method (8). In both cases the iodinated antibody, R9.75, was injected into nontumor-bearing nude mice (control) as well as into nude mice that had been inoculated with BN lymphoma cells. Table 4 shows the tissue-to-blood ratios 24 h after injection of the direct- and oligosaccharide-linked antibodies into both control and tumor-bearing mice. Despite an equivalent degree of immunoreactivity for both preparations (89% and 85% for the direct- and oligosaccharide-linked antibodies, respectively), there was substantially greater tumor localization in animals injected with the oligosaccharide-linked conjugate than in those injected with the directly iodinated antibody. In addition, the oligosaccharide-linked conjugate localized in the liver to a greater extent than did the direct-linked conjugate. From other experiments in this tumor system we have determined that the tumor metastasizes; we believe that these metastases are going to the liver. In neither group of control mice was nonspecific localization evident for any tissue, including the liver.

Another interesting finding in this experiment was the higher circulating levels of the radioactive dose in animals injected with the site-specific modified conjugate. Twenty-four hours after administration, only 19.3% of the total injected dose was retained in the tissues examined from mice injected with the directly iodinated antibody; in contrast, 83% of the total injected dose was retained in mice injected with the oligosaccharide-linked antibody. Ultimately these higher circulating levels may be of therapeutic importance.

Table 5 Considerations in Selecting an Isotope
for Radiotherapy

Physical half-life

Gamma energies and abundances

Particle radiation

Efficiency of particle versus photon radiation

Specific activity

Metal ion contamination

Stability of radionuclide-proton bond

Production of radioisotope

IV. RADIOIMMUNOTHERAPEUTIC STUDIES WITH 212-BISMUTH AND 90-YTTRIUM

In selecting a radioisotope with potential therapeutic utility, we focused on chelatable metals since our site-specific modification process with GYK-DTPA had worked well with ^{111}In. After consideration of the physical properties, potential therapeutic advantages, and production feasibility of several isotopes, we selected two chelatable metals for further evaluation: ^{212}Bi, an alpha emitter, and ^{90}Y, a beta emitter. In this section, our considerations in selecting these radioisotopes are first outlined and then preliminary data in tumor-bearing mice using antibody conjugates labeled with these two metals are reviewed.

A. Considerations in Selecting a Radioisotope

Table 5 lists our considerations in selecting isotopes for radiotherapy. Any isotope considered should have a sufficiently long physical half-life to enable it to localize at the desired tumor site and exert its therapeutic activity. The two

Table 6 Radiolysis of Labeled Antibodies

Isotope	Specific activity (μCi/μg)	Time (h)	Percent Immunoreactivity −BSA	+BSA
^{212}Bi	14	24	100	100
^{90}Y	50	24	100	100
	110	24	65	76
	110	48	37	70

Abbreviation: BSA = bovine serum albumin.

isotopes we selected represent extremes of physical half-lives; ^{212}Bi has a 1-h half-life while ^{90}Y has a 64-h half-life. We also selected two radioisotopes with different particle energies. Alpha particles are very cytotoxic but have a short kill radius, 50-80 μm. As a result, only cells that immediately surround an antibody coupled to an alpha emitter such as ^{212}Bi will be killed. These properties are very desirable if the tumor is highly localized and if the destruction of surrounding, nontumor-bearing cells is unacceptable. 90-Yttrium, on the other hand, is a beta emitter which has a larger radius of cytotoxic activity but is less potent than ^{212}Bi.

The specific activity is a measure of the amount of nonradioactive isotope present in the preparation, and as such has a direct bearing on its potential therapeutic utility. For example, if the specific activity of a metal isotope is too low, then the amount which ultimately becomes attached to an antibody may be too little to provide any therapeutic benefit. For ^{111}In a specific activity of 2 to 5 μCi/μg is adequate for imaging in mice and humans. In our laboratory, the typical range of specific activity for ^{212}Bi is 1 to 5 μCi/μg, although we are trying to increase it beyond this. We have steadily increased the specific activity of ^{90}Y from 10 to 50 μCi/μg to 200 μCi/μg as the quality of the yttrium supply has increased. Interestingly, we have found that as the specific activity increases, the potential for radiolysis also increases. As shown in Table 6, when the specific activity of ^{90}Y was increased to 110 μCi/μg, immunoreactivity decreased from 100% at zero hours to 65% and 37% at 24 and 48 h, respectively. We could retard the degree of radiolysis somewhat by adding a protein, bovine serum albumin (BSA), to the incubation solution. No radiolysis was evident when the specific activities of ^{212}Bi and ^{90}Y were 14 and 50 μCi/μg, respectively.

Metal ion contamination, even in trace amounts, can result in low incorporation of the isotope. For example, using a technique for extracting indium from other metal ions (15), we have been able to increase the specific activity of antibodies labeled with ^{111}In to 180 μCi/μg.

The stability of the radionuclide-protein bond is of obvious importance as a radioisotope has little utility for immunotherapy or immunoscintigraphy if it is not possible to chelate the isotope or to form a strong bond with the antibody.

The physical and economic feasibility of producing prospective isotopes is also a factor in selecting a candidate. The bismuth generator we use was developed at Argonne National Laboratories and is diagrammed in Figure 6. The generator starts with 228-Thorium and the ^{212}Bi eventually decays to stable lead. Because of the relatively short half-life of ^{212}Bi, we explored the possibility of attaching its immediate precursor, 212-lead, to the antibody because it has a longer half-life. Unfortunately, GYK-DTPA does not chelate 212-lead. The yttrium we use is generated from 90-strontium (Fig. 7), which has a 28.5 year half-life. The 90-yttrium eventually decays to stable 90-zirconium.

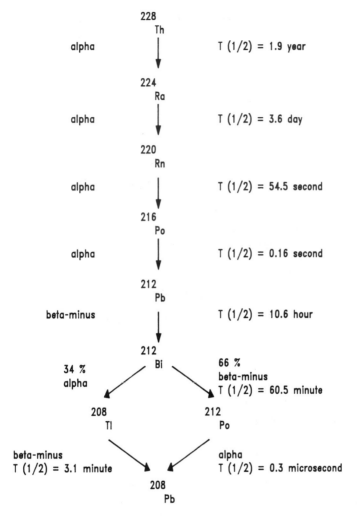

Figure 6   Decay scheme of ^{212}Bi generator used to produce ^{212}Bi.

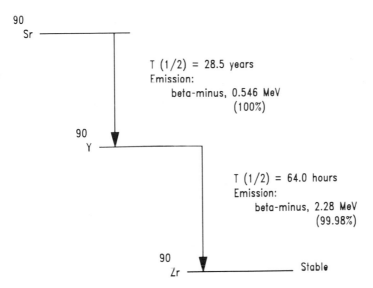

Figure 7 Decay scheme of ^{90}Sr used to produce ^{90}Y.

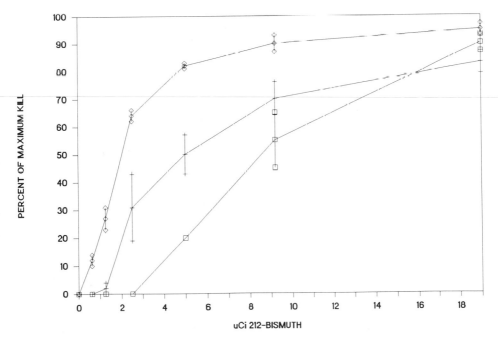

Figure 8 In vitro cytotoxic effect of ^{212}Bi-labeled B72.3 monoclonal antibody in LS174T cell line. Percent maximum killing due to ^{212}Bi alone (□), ^{212}Bi-labeled irrelevant antibody (+), or ^{212}Bi-labeled B72.3 (specific antibody) (◇).

B. Cytotoxic Activity of 212-Bismuth-Labeled Antibodies

In evaluating the therapeutic potential of ^{212}Bi and ^{90}Y we used the LS174T cell line. This cell line originated from a colon carcinoma xenograft and was chosen, in part, because it is moderately radioresistant. Any therapeutic effects achieved with this target would suggest at least similar effects in more radiosensitive systems. Another advantage to the LS174T cell line is its high antigen content which provides an opportunity for large amounts of the antibody conjugate to localize to the tumor site. The monoclonal antibody used, B72.3, is an IgG obtained in response to human adenocarcinoma; it has a high crossreactivity to many different mucin-producing tumors, including those localized in the ovaries, breast and colon.

In a preliminary in vitro study in the LS174T cell line, we compared the cytotoxic effects of the ^{212}Bi-labeled B72.3 antibody, ^{212}Bi alone and a ^{212}Bi labeled antibody not specific for the LS174T cell line. The two antibodies were labeled to a specific activity of 5 μCi/μg and were incubated in various dilutions of ^{212}Bi. As shown in Figure 8, the cytotoxic effects of the three treatment conditions were similar at an activity of 19-20 μCi ^{212}Bi and the percent of LS174T target cells killed approached 100%. At lower activities, differences among the three groups emerged. At activities between 1 and 10 μCi of ^{212}Bi, the cytotoxic activity of the ^{212}Bi-labeled B72.3 antibody was substantially greater than that of the ^{212}Bi-labeled nonspecific antibody or of ^{212}Bi alone. We are continuing to explore this immunospecific cytotoxicity with ^{212}Bi against the LS174T cell line by varying both the specific activity of the isotope and the incubation interval. Even with relatively short incubation intervals, we have been able to demonstrate immunospecific cytotoxicity with ^{212}Bi.

In our in vitro experiments with ^{212}Bi the GYK-DTPA chelator-radioisotope attachment was quite stable. A different picture emerged when we administered the ^{212}Bi-labeled antibody in vivo. Within 5 minutes following intravenous injection of the ^{212}Bi-labeled GYK-DTPA antibody conjugate to normal mice, there was measurable radioactivity in the kidney. Biodistribution determinations performed 1 h after injection of the ^{212}Bi-labeled antibody showed percent injected dose per gram (%I.D./g) values in the kidneys as high as 100% I.D./g. As shown in Table 7, comparable values for ^{111}In-labeled antibodies are 11% I.D./g; these data indicate that the ^{212}Bi must be stripped from the chelate by the kidneys. This level of recovery for ^{111}In remained essentially constant over time (data not shown in Table 7), but it increased for ^{212}Bi 2 h after intravenous administration. As expected, injecting the radiolabeled antibody intraperitoneally (i.p.) retarded the rate of uptake in the kidney. One hour after i.p. administration of ^{212}Bi-labeled GYK-DTPA antibody conjugate only 20% I.D./g was present in the kidney; however, after four hours, 117% I.D./g was evident in the kidney.

Table 7 In Vivo Stability of 111-Indium and 212-Bismuth: Activity in the Kidney

Route of administration	Time after administration (h)	Percent I.D./g	
		[111]In	[212]Bi
Intravenous	1	11.2	100.1
	2	–	121.6
Intraperitoneal	1	4.0	20.4
	2	–	48.6
	4	–	117.0

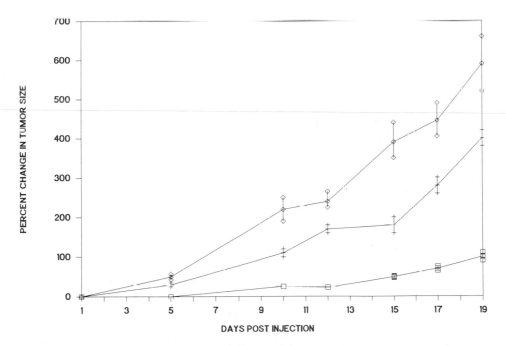

Figure 9 In vivo cytotoxic effect of ^{90}Y-labeled B72.3 monoclonal antibody in LS174T tumor xenografts. Percent change in tumor size after two injections of unlabeled B72.3 (◊), ^{90}Y-labeled irrelevant antibody (+), or ^{90}Y-labeled B72.3 (specific antibody) (□).

These data clearly demonstrate that there is preferential uptake by the kidney of ^{212}Bi when it is linked to an antibody via the chelator GYK-DTPA. The potential for nephrotoxicity following the use of ^{212}Bi can be diminished if the radioisotope is administered i.p. because by the time of substantial accumulation, the isotope has decayed. We are currently evaluating other chelators for ^{212}Bi in an attempt to further reduce the uptake of this radioisotope by the kidney.

C. Cytotoxic Activity of ^{90}Y-Labeled Antibodies

The therapeutic effect of ^{90}Y-labeled B72.3 antibody conjugate on the LS174T cell line was evaluated in vivo in our laboratory. Nude mice were injected with the LS174T cell line in the left flank seven days prior to treatment. In preliminary studies, intravenous administration of a single 200 μCi dose of ^{90}Y-labeled B72.3 antibody was lethal to the mice while a single 100 μCi dose failed to have any discernable effect on tumor growth. When we administered two 100 μCi doses of ^{90}Y-labeled B72.3 antibody, each dose separated by one day, tumor growth was significantly retarded (Fig. 9). In both the control mice (injected with the incubation solution only) and mice given two injections of a ^{90}Y-labeled antibody not specific for the LS174T cell line, the tumor continued to grow throughout the 20-day observation period. At the end of the 20-day post-dose period, there was some increase in the tumor size for animals treated with ^{90}Y-labeled B72.3 antibody. It is possible that this growth could have been inhibited had additional injections been administered during the 20-day period. Indeed, subsequent studies in our laboratory have shown that multiple injections given at appropriate intervals will virtually retard tumor growth in this experimental model.

V. SUMMARY AND CONCLUSIONS

Site-specific covalent modification of monoclonal antibodies at the oligosaccharide offers advantages over more conventional modification processes that involve direct attachment at tyrosine, lysine or glutamic/aspartic acid side chains. Using the site-specific modification process, attachment sites on the antibody are distal to the antigen-binding region. Thus, homogeneity of antigen-binding properties and affinity for the unmodified protein are preserved. Furthermore, higher derivatization ratios with no resultant loss of immunoreactivity can be achieved for monoclonal antibodies modified at the oligosaccharide.

In vivo biodistribution and tumor localization studies in nude mouse models suggest that antibodies radiolabeled at their oligosaccharide might represent improved immunoscintigraphic reagents. In a variety of tumor xenograft models, site-specific modified ^{111}In-labeled antibody conjugates localized to the tumor site with little non-specific localization in other tissues or organs. The degree of localization at the target site was substantially greater than that of ^{111}In-labeled antibodies directly modified at the tyrosine side chain.

Preliminary studies with ^{212}Bi- and ^{90}Y-labeled antibodies modified at the oligosaccharide indicate that both of these radioisotopes have immunotherapeutic potential. Because of its preferential uptake by the kidney, the use of ^{212}Bi may be best suited for tumors localized within the peritoneal cavity, such as ovarian and colorectal carcinomas. The toxicity of ^{90}Y at high specific activities suggests that a regimen of repeated smaller doses of this radioisotope is best suited for therapeutic use. Studies in tumor-bearing mouse models are currently underway to better define the optimal dosage and administration regimens for both of these radioisotopes when attached to site-specific modified antibodies.

ACKNOWLEDGMENTS

The authors would like to acknowledge the excellent technical skills of Grace Greway, Ann Blake, Kurt Richau, and Judy Hauler. We would also like to thank Angelica Alarcon for her excellent secretarial help.

REFERENCES

1. Kohler, G., and Milstein C. (1975). Continuous cultures of fused cells secreting antibody of predefined specificity. *Nature 256*:495–497.
2. Mach, J. P., Carrel, S., Forni, M., Ritxchard, J., Donath, A., and Alberto, P. (1980). Tumor localization of radiolabeled antibodies to carcinoembryonic antigen for the detection and localization of diverse cancers by external photoscanning. *New Engl. J. Med. 300*:5–10.
3. Rainsbury, R. M., Westwood, J. H., Coombes, R. C., Neville, A. M., Ott, R. J., Kalirai, T. S., McCready, V. R., and Gazet, J. C. (1983). Localization of metastatic breast carcinoma by a Mab chelate labelled with indium-111. *Lancet ii*:934–938.
4. Epenetos, A. A., Britton, K. E., Mather, S., Shepherd, J., Granowska, M., Taylor-Papadimitriou, J., Nimmon, C. C., Durbin, H., Hawkins, L. R., Malpas, J. S., and Bodmer, W. F. (1982). Targeting of iodine-123-labelled tumor-associated monoclonal antibodies to ovarian, breast and gastrointestinal tumors. *Lancet ii*:999–1005.
5. Baldwin, R. W., Embleton, M. J., and Pimm, M. V. (1982). Monoclonal antitumor antibodies for tumor detection and therapy. *Bull. Cancer 70*:103–107.
6. Youle, R. J., and Neville, D. M. (1980). Anti-Thy 1.2 monoclonal antibody linked to ricin is a potent cell-type-specific toxin. *Proc. Natl. Acad. Sci. USA 77*:5483–5486.
7. Alvarez, V. L., Lopes, A. D., Lee, C., Coughlin, D. J., Rodwell, J. D., and McKearn, T. J. (1988). Site-specific modification of monoclonal antibodies:

studies of 111-Indium labeled antibodies using nude mouse xenograft systems. In *Antibody Mediated Delivery Systems*. Edited by J. D. Rodwell. Marcel Dekker, New York, pp. 283–315.

8. Rodwell, J. D., Alvarez, V. L., Lee, C., Lopes, A. D., Goers, J. W. F., King, H. D., Powsner, H. J., and McKearn, T. J. (1986). Site-specific covalent modification of monoclonal antibodies. *In vitro* and *in vivo* evaluations. *Proc. Natl. Acad. Sci. USA 83*:2632–2636.

9. Goodwin, D. A., Meares, C. F., McCall, M. J., Haseman, M. K., McTigue, M., Dimanti, C.I., and Chaovapang, W. (1985). Chelate conjugates of monoclonal antibodies for imaging lymphoid structures in the mouse. *J. Nucl. Med. 26*:493–502.

10. Paik, C. H., Hong, J. J., Ebbert, M. A., Heald, S. C., Reba, R. C., and Eckelman, W. C. (1985). Relative reactivity of DTPA, immunoreactive antibody-DTPA conjugates, and non-immunoreactive antibody-DTPA conjugates toward indium-111. *J. Nucl. Med. 26*:482–487.

11. Hnatowich, D. J., Layne, W. W., Childs, R. L., Lantegne, D., Davis, M. A., Griffin, T. W., and Doherty, P. W. (1983). Radioactive labeling of antibody: A simple and efficient method. *Science 220*:613–615.

12. Halpern, J. E., Hagan, P. L., and Garver, P. R. (1984). Stability, characterization and kinetics of 111-In-labeled monoclonal anti-tumor antibodies in normal animals and nude mouse-human tumor models. *J. Can. Res. 43*: 5347–5355.

13. Perkins, A. C., Pimm, M. V., and Birch, M. K. (1985). The preparation and characterization of 111-In-labeled 7915/36 monoclonal antibody for tumor immunoscintigraphy. *Eur. J. Nucl. Med. 10*:296–301.

14. Alvarez, V. L., Wen, M., Lee, C., Lopes, A. D., Rodwell, J. D., and McKearn, T. J. (1986). Site-specifically modified 111-Indium labeled antibodies give low liver backgrounds and improved radioimmunoscintigraphy. *Nucl. Med. Biol. 13*:347–352.

15. Zoghbi, S. S., Neumann, R. D., and Gotschalk, A. (1986). The ultrapurification of indium-111 for radiotracer studies. *Invest. Radiol. 21*:710–713.

6

Killing of Human Tumor Cells by Antibody C3b Conjugates and Human Complement

YORAM REITER and ZVI FISHELSON
The Weizmann Institute of Science, Rehovot, Israel

I. INTRODUCTION

The activation of the alternative pathway of complement commences by a covalent attachment of C3b molecules to the surface of complement activators (1). Factor B binds in the presence of magnesium ions to this C3b and is then cleaved by Factor D thus yielding the C3 convertase C3b,Bb (1-4). This enzyme, by cleaving C3 to C3b, effects further deposition of C3b molecules on activating surfaces and thereby generation of surface-bound C3/C5 convertases, which cleave C5 molecules to C5b and initiate the generation of the membrane attack complex of complement, C5b-9 (5). The number of surface-bound C3b molecules is regulated by Factors H and I (6-10); Factor H restricts the formation of the C3 convertase by competing with Factor B binding and accelerates the decay-dissociation of the C3 convertase into its two subunits C3b and Bb. Furthermore, Factor H serves as a cofactor in the proteolytic degradation of C3b molecules by Factor I (8-10).

Nucleated cells and in particular tumor cells are more resistant to complement-mediated killing than red blood cells (11,12). This is probably due either to membrane regulatory molecules which reduce the number of surface-bound C3b molecules and/or membrane attack complexes on the target cells (13–15) or to defense mechanisms which are employed by the nucleated cells to repair a complement-mediated damage (16). The monoclonal antibody technology (17) have opened new perspectives in immunotherapy as they permit the targeting of toxins or drug selectivity to the antigen-bearing cell population (18). Others have attempted to target the complement system to specific cells by using conjugates composed of the C3b-like glycoprotein of cobra verum (cobra verum factor, CVF) and antibodies (19,20). The CVF was directed by a monoclonal antibody to a human melanoma-associated antigen (19) or to human erythrocytes (20) and potentiated complement killing of these target cells. We describe herewith the generation and characterization of a different heteroconjugate which can potentiate the lytic action of homologous complement on tumor cells. This heteroconjugate is composed of a murine monoclonal antibody and of the human C3b complement component (mAb-C3b). The antibody which was used is transferrin receptor-specific monoclonal antibody. The obligatory expression of these receptors during growth and their abundancy on tumor cells relative to normal tissues (21,22) makes them good targets for experimental immunotherapy.

II. MATERIALS AND METHODS

A. Complement Proteins and Buffers

Complement components C3 and Factors H and I were isolated from human plasma as previously described (23) and C3b was generated from C3 by trypsin cleavage (24). C3b was then purified over Sephacryl S-300 column (Pharmacia, Uppsala, Sweden). Proteins were radiolabeled with ^{125}I (Amersham, Arlington Heights, IL) by the Iodogen method (25) (Pierce Chemical Co., Roxford, IL). Experiments were carried out in phosphate-buffered saline (0.15 M), pH 7.4 containing 0.02% sodium azide (PBS).

B. Cells and Monoclonal Antibody

The K562 human myelogenous leukemia (26) was kept in culture in RPMI-1640 (Gibco Laboratories, Grand Island, NY) supplemented with 10% (v/v) heat-inactivated fetal calf serum, penicillin (100 U/ml), streptomycin (0.4 mg/ml), and fungizon (0.02 mg/ml) (Bio-Lab, Jerusalem, Israel). The V1-10 hybridoma (obtained from Dr. Zelig Eshhar) was kept in Dulbecco's modified Eagle medium (Gibco), supplemented with 10% (v/v) heat-inactivated fetal calf serum, and antibiotic mixture as above. The V1-10 monoclonal antibody (IgG$_1$) was isolated from ascites fluid of BALB/c $\times$ C57BL/6 F1 mice using a protein A-Sepharose 4B (Pharmacia) column.

C. Generation of mAb-C3b Conjugates: Crosslinking with Glutaraldehyde

Glutaraldehyde (10%) was added to a solution of ^{125}I-labeled C3b (175 μg) and V1-10 mAb (175 μg) in PBS, pH 7.4, to give final concentration of 0.3 or 1%. Titration of the pH to 9.5 was performed by addition of concentrated carbonate buffer (0.1M, pH 9.6). The mixture was incubated at 20°C for 30 min and the reaction was stopped by adding 2M glycine, pH 8.0 (Sigma) or 2M lysine, pH 8.2 (Merck) to a final concentration of 0.2M. Excess reagent was removed from the protein mixture by centrifugation through a Biogel P-6 column (Bio-Rad Labs, Richmond, CA).

D. Crosslinking with SPDP

Conjugation was performed as previously described (19,27) by thiol-disulfide exchange using the heterobifunctional reagent N-succinimidyl-3-(2-pyridyldithio) propionate (SPDP, Pierce Chemical Co., Rockford, IL). SPDP (20mM) in absolute ethanol was added to C3b or monoclonal antibody (0.5 mg each) in PBS to give a 5.5 molar excess of SPDP/protein. Each protein was stirred at room temperature for 30 min and then gel filtered over a column of Sephadex G-25 medium (Pharmacia). The pyridyldithiopropionylated monoclonal antibody in 0.1M sodium acetate, 0.1M NaCl, pH 4.5, was reduced with 45mM dithiothreitol (Bio Rad) for 20 min at room temperature and then gel filtered over Sephadex G-25. The thiolated antibody was immediately mixed for cross-linking with equimolar amounts of pyridyldithiopropionylated C3b and incubated for 24 hours at room temperature. The protein mixture was then gel filtered at 4°C over a Sephacryl S-300 column and peak fractions were analyzed by sodium dodecylsulfate (SDS)-polyacrylamide gel electrophoresis on 5% gels.

E. Cytotoxicity and Binding Assay

K562 cells (5×10^5) were exposed to serum for various time periods at 37°C as indicated. Alternatively, cells were incubated for 30 min on ice with antibodies or antibody-C3b conjugates, washed three times with PBS, and then incubated at 37°C with 100 μl normal human serum diluted 1/2 with PBS. Cytolysis was determined microscopically by dye exclusion with 0.1% (w/v) trypan blue (Fluka AG, Buchs, SG, Switzerland). To measure antibody or antibody-C3b conjugate binding, K562 cells (10^6) were incubated with ^{125}I-labeled protein in 100 μl PBS for 90 min on ice. The unbound protein was then removed by centrifugation through 20% sucrose in 0.4 ml polyethylene microtest tubes (Bio-Rad). Nonspecific binding was determined by addition of 20-fold excess of unlabeled protein.

F. SDS-PAGE and Immunoelectrophoresis

SDS-polyacrylamide gel electrophoresis was performed according to Laemmli (28) on 5% or 10% slab gels. Proteins were analyzed by immunoelectrophoresis in 1.2% (w/v) agarose LE (FMC Co., Richmond, CA) in Tris-glycine buffer, pH 8.6. Washed and dried gels were stained with amido black (Bio-Rad) (0.05% in 40% ethanol, 10% glacial acetic acid in H_2O).

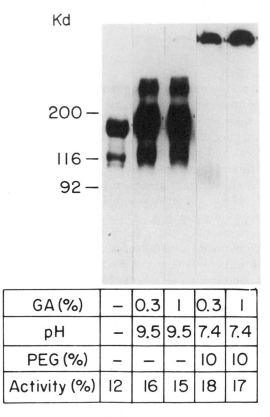

GA (%)	–	0.3	1	0.3	1
pH	–	9.5	9.5	7.4	7.4
PEG (%)	–	–	–	10	10
Activity (%)	12	16	15	18	17

Figure 1 Cross-linking of V1-10 mAb and C3b with glutaraldehyde. V1-10 mAb and ^{125}I-labelled C3b were cross-linked as explained under Materials and Methods. The reaction products were analyzed by SDS-PAGE on 5% gels which were dried and subjected to autoradiography. To measure the complement-promoting activity of the conjugates, 5×10^5 K562 cells were incubated with the cross-linking products for 60 min at 4°C, washed, and then incubated for 90 min at 37°C with normal human serum diluted 1/2 in PBS. Percent cytolysis (% activity) was determined by trypan blue exclusion.

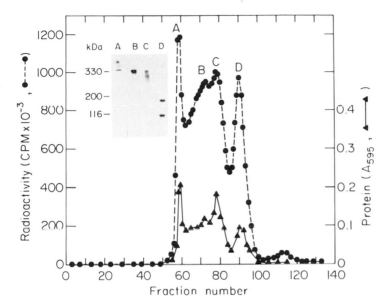

Figure 2 Gel filtration of V1-10 mAb-C3b conjugates following cross-linking with SPDP. The reaction mixture of ^{125}I-labelled C3b and V1-10 mAb following cross-linking with SPDP was applied to a Sephacryl S-300 column. Peak fractions A–D were analyzed on 5% SDS-PAGE. Radiographs of peak fractions are shown in the insert.

III. RESULTS AND DISCUSSION

A. Preparation and Isolation of mAb-C3b Heteroconjugates

C3b was covalently linked to the murine monoclonal antibody using two different methods: glutaraldehyde or SPDP cross-linking. In the first approach, ^{125}I-labeled C3b and V1-10 mAb were reacted in the presence of glutaraldehyde at pH 7.4 or 9.5. This produced almost no conjugates. However, upon addition of polyethylenglycol (10%) into the reaction mixture, a closer contact was induced between the C3b and antibody molecules and the conjugation was successful, yielding a major product of about 340,000 dalton (Fig. 1). Unfortunately, the complement-promoting activity of glutaraldehyde-derived complexes was very low. Only 3–6% increase in killing of K562 by normal human serum was observed when glutaraldehyde-derived V1-10-C3b conjugates were added. This failure to activate the complement cascade on K562 cells could be due to inactivation of C3b or to inhibition of the antibody-binding activity by glutaraldehyde.

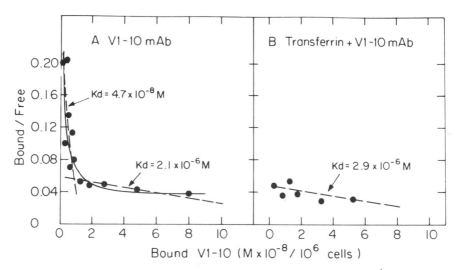

Figure 3 Scatchard plot of the binding of V1-10 mAb to K562: 10^6 cells were
incubated for 60 min at $0°C$ with or without 100 μg transferrin. The cells were
then washed and incubated for 90 min at $4°C$ with various concentrations of
^{125}I-labelled V1-10 mAb. Binding was quantitated as described under Materials
and Methods.

However, using the heterobifunctional reagend SPDP, stable and active mAb-
C3b conjugates could be produced. Thiolated antibody and SPDP-treated C3b
were mixed and incubated for 24 h (for further details, see Materials and Methods). The mixture was then subjected to gel filtration on a Sephacryl S-300
column. As shown in Figure 2, the protein was resolved into four peaks (A–D).
SDS-PAGE analysis of peak fractions revealed the presence of conjugates as well
as free C3b. The major conjugate species (lanes B) had a molecular weight of
about 330,000, which corresponds to a complex of one antibody and one C3b.
This conjugate was subsequently found to be a highly active promoter of complement-mediated killing of tumor cells.

B. Binding of the mAb-C3b Conjugates to K562

The monoclonal antibody used in this study is directed to the transferrin receptor which is highly expressed on the surface of malignant cells. K562 cells express approximately 6×10^5 transferrin receptors per cell and bind the V1-10
mAb with a Kd of about $5 \times 10^{-8} M$ (Fig. 3). Analysis of the V1-10 mAb binding
to K562 cells by the indirect immunofluorescence technique demonstrated that
all of the cells bind the antibody (not shown). A biphasic Scatchard plot of

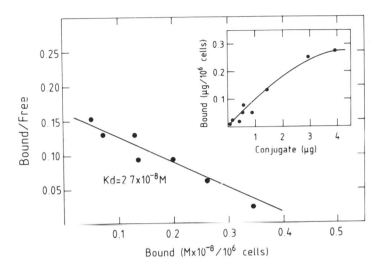

Figure 4 Binding of V1-10 mAb-C3b conjugates to K562 cells: 10^6 cells were incubated for 90 min at 4°C with various concentrations of ^{125}I-labeled conjugates. Binding was quantitated as described under Materials and Methods. The binding curve (insert) and Scatchard plot analysis are presented.

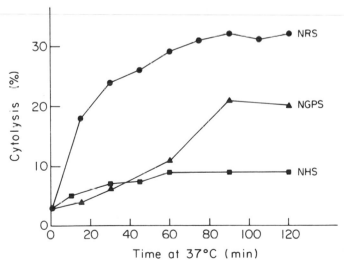

Figure 5 Lysis of K562 by normal rabbit, guinea pig or human sera: 5×10^5 cells were incubated for different times at 37°C with 100 μl normal rabbit (NRS), guinea pig (NGPS), or human (NHS) sera diluted 1/2 in PBS.

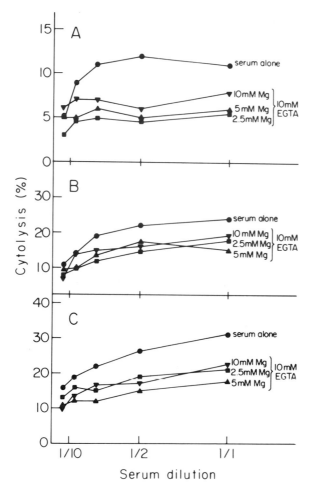

Figure 6 Effect of MgEGTA on killing of K562 by normal human, guinea pig, or rabbit sera: 5×10^5 cells were incubated for 60 min at $37°C$ with 100 μl normal human (NHS), guinea pig (NGPS), or rabbit (NRS) sera containing Mg^{2+} and EGTA at concentrations indicated.

V1-10 mAb binding to K562 revealed that the binding involves two sites, one with a high and one with a low affinity. Pretreatment of the K562 cells with transferrin prior to antibody binding blocked the high affinity binding and had no effect on the low affinity binding. This suggests that the antibody binds with a high affinity ($5 \times 10^{-8}M$) to the transferrin receptor and with a low affinity ($2 \times 10^{-6}M$) to yet another receptor on the cell surface, probably the Fc receptor.

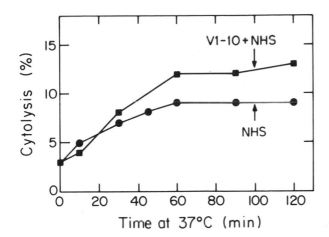

Figure 7 Lysis of K562 by V1-10 mAb and normal human serum: 5×10^5 cells were incubated for 30 min at $4°C$ with or without 125 µg V1-10 mAb in 100 µl PBS. Following washing the cells were incubated with 100 µl normal human serum diluted 1/2 in PBS at $37°C$. Percent lysis was determined at various times by trypan blue exclusion.

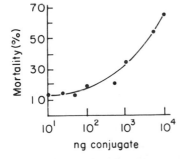

Experiment	Conjugates (µg)			
	5	10	20	30
	(percent mortality)			
1	53	67	69	69
2	51	68	69	70

Figure 8 Lysis of K562 cells by V1-10 mAb-C3b conjugates and normal human serum: 5×10^5 cells were incubated for 60 min at $4°C$ with various concentratins of V-10 mAb-C3b conjugates, washed, and further incubated for 90 min at $37°C$ with normal human serum diluted 1/2 in PBS.

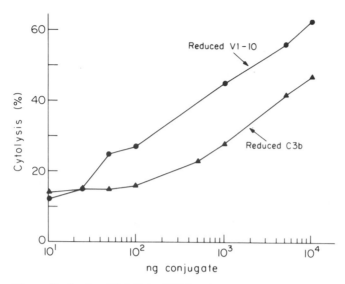

Figure 9 Lysis of K562 by NHS and conjugates prepared with thiolated V1-10 mAb or thiolated C3b: 5×10^6 cells were incubated for 60 min at 37°C with conjugates made with either reduced C3b or reduced V1-10 mAb. The cells were then washed and further incubated for 60 min at 37°C with 100 μl NHS diluted 1/2 in PBS.

The C3b-conjugated V1-10 mAb bound to K562 cells with a similar affinity $(2.7 \times 10^{-8} M)$ but lacked the low affinity phase of the Scatchard curve (Fig. 4). This may indicate that the cross-linked C3b is sterically blocking the Fc receptor binding site of the mAb or that the cross-linking procedure modified this site in the antibody.

C. Potentiation of Tumor Cell Killing with mAb-C3b Conjugates

Tumor cells, or nucleated cells in general, are known to vary in their susceptibility to complement-mediated killing (12,16). Thus, for example, K562 cells are rather resistant to complement-mediated killing in absence of added antibodies in homologous human serum but less so in heterologous sera (Fig. 5). This phenomenon of homologous species restriction in lysis by complement has previously been demonstrated in other systems (15,29). Activation of the classical pathway of complement requires both Ca^{2+} and Mg^{2+} ions whereas only Mg^{2+} ions are required for alternative pathway activation (30). Mg-EGTA, which selectively removes Ca^{2+}, enables measurements of alternative pathway activation in whole serum. Figure 6 shows the effect of Mg-EGTA on killing of K562 by

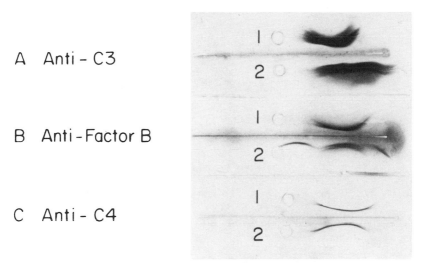

A   Anti - C3

B   Anti - Factor B

C   Anti - C4

I - NHS control

2 - Conjugate-treated NHS

Figure 10 Activation of the alternative pathway of complement by V1-10 mAb-C3b conjugates. V1-10 mAb-C3b conjugates were mixed with normal human serum for 90 min at 37°C. Serum aliquots were then analyzed by immunoelectrophoresis using goat anti-human C3, Factor B, and C4 antibodies.

normal human, guinea pig, and rabbit sera. The partial decrease in killing observed in presence of Mg-EGTA indicates that the K562 cells activate both the classical and alternative pathways of complement in the three sera which were studied. The molecules which activate complement on K562 cells, being surface membrane molecules and/or natural antibodies which occur in normal human guinea pig, and rabbit sera, are not yet defined. As shown in Figure 7, the V1-10 mAb is a poor activator of complement and pretreatment of the cells with the antibody increased only slightly (from 9 to 13%) the lysis of K562 cells by normal human serum. However, following pretreatment of K562 cells with the V1-10 mAb-C3b conjugates and incubation with normal human serum, cell lysis increased to about 70% (Fig. 8). A similar conjugation efficiency was obtained whether thiolated C3b or thiolated antibody were used during the crosslinking procedure. However, as shown in Figure 9, conjgates made with thiolated C3b promoted less killing of K562 cells by normal human serum as compared with conjugates made with thiolated antibody. The effect of the conjugate was

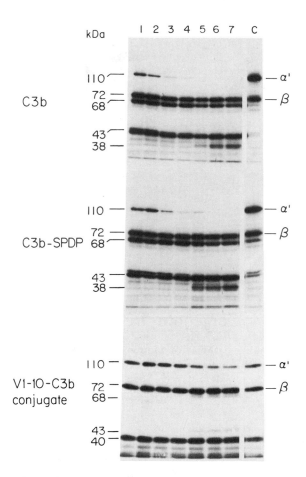

Figure 11 Cleavage of C3b, C3b-SPDP, and conjugated-C3b by Factors H and I. C3b, SPDP-treated C3b, or V1-10 mAb-C3b conjugates (^{125}I-labeled C3b) were incubated for 90 min at 37°C with various concentrations of Factors H and I. The samples were reduced and analyzed on 10% gels by SDS-PAGE. The gels were dried and exposed to autoradiography. Lane 1: 0.5 μg Factor H, 0.05 μg Factor 1; lane 2: 1, 0.1; lane 3: 2, 0.2; lane 4: 4, 04; lane 5: 8, 0.8; lane 6: 16, 1.6; lane 7: 32, 3.2; C: Control without Factors H and I.

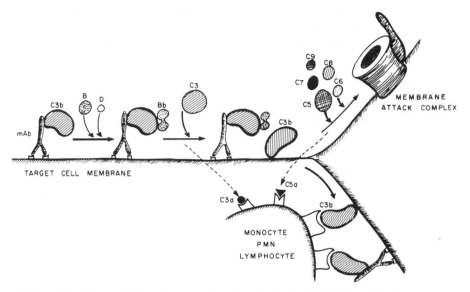

Figure 12 The activities of monoclonal antibody (mAb)-C3b conjugates. Schematic representation of the various immunological processes which may follow binding of mAb-C3b conjugates to tumor cells.

dose dependent, however, conjugate input of 10 μg per 10^6 cells and higher could not increase K562 cell killing to above 70%. At the same time, almost 100% killing of BALB/c lymphoma ALB1 cells could be induced by a similar mAb-C3b conjugate which was directed to the murine transferrin receptor and normal human serum (data not shown). These results demonstrate that the K562 cell population is heterogenic in its sensitivity to complement killing. Recently, by repeatedly exposing the K562 cells to conjugate and complement treatments we could select for a subline which is completely resistant to killing by conjugates and serum. This complement-resistant subline of K562 binds the same number of antibody molecules as the parental line (31).

D. Interactions of the mAb-C3b Conjugates with the Alternative Pathway of Complement

Coupling of C3b to the monoclonal antibody apparently converted it to an activator of the complement system. Indeed, when such conjugates were introduced into normal human serum which was then incubated at 37°C, a dose-dependent activation and consumption of complement occurred. To determine whether the mAb-C3b conjugates activate the classical or alternative pathway, the fate of the complement components C3, Factor B, and C4 in the activated serum was studied. The immunoelectrophoretic migration patterns of these proteins (Fig. 10) demonstrated that C3 and Factor B were cleaved during the activation by mAb-C3b conjugates, whereas C4 was not affected. This is indicative of a selective activation of the alternative pathway of complement.

C3b molecules which are generated during complement activation in serum are usually rapidly inactivated by Factors H and I. Therefore, such an efficient activation of complement by mAb-C3b conjugates was not expected. To determine how sensitive is the conjugated C3b to regulation, it was incubated with purified Factors H and I and then analyzed by SDS-PAGE. Native and SPDP-treated C3b served as control. C3b is composed of α' and β chains. Following inactivation by Factors H and I, the α' chain is degraded to 68,000 and 43,000 Mr fragments. As shown in Figure 11, both native C3b and SPDP-treated C3b were efficiently degraded by Factors H and I. On the other hand, conjugated C3b was much more stable and was only partially inactivated even by high concentration of Factors H and I (Fig. 11, lane 7). This resistance of conjugated C3b to inactivation results probably from its reduced Factor H binding capacity (not shown).

E. Concluding Remarks

Heteroconjugates composed of antitumor antibodies and of C3b are hereby proposed to be efficient tools which can activate complement on selected cells. As a model system we have used monoclonal antibodies to transferrin receptor. However, the specificity and selectivity of action of such conjugates will soon be examined with monoclonal antibodies to specific or unique tumor antigens. By coupling C3b to such antibodies it is possible now to convert any monoclonal antibody to a complement activator rather than being limited to the small fraction of monoclonal antibodies which are naturally activating complement. As was earlier proposed, a similar result may be obtained by coupling the cobra venom factor to antibodies (19,20). Cobra venom factor generates the C3/C5 convertase more efficiently than C3b. However, when considering the application of mAb-CVF or mAb-C3b conjugates for in vivo therapy, CVF will probably be highly immunogenic in humans and its activity will be limited to one or two treatments. Another advantage of using conjugates containing C3b but not CVF is the postulated activity which mAb-C3b but not mAb-CVF conjugates will have in potentiating the cytotoxic activity of leukocytes and lymphocytes on selected target cells. As presented schematically in Figure 12, the target cell-conjugated C3b will produce three responses: (1) amplification of C3b deposition and generation of membrane attack complexes. (2) generation of the chemotactic and inflammatory complement peptides C3a and C5a which can also induce increased vascular permeability (32); and (3) attachment of C3 receptor-positive leukocytes (32,33) and possibly activation of their cytotoxic mechanisms. Combined, these effector mechanisms which may be activated in vivo by antitumor antibodies coupled to C3b and specifically directed to the tumor cells, may facilitate tumor immunotherapy. The in vivo potency of mAb-C3b conjugates is being now tested in several experimental tumor models.

IV. SUMMARY

To potentiate the lytic action of complement on tumor cells, we have constructed heteroconjugates composed of monoclonal antibody and of the human C3b component of complement. The conjugates were formed efficiently using the heterobifunctional cross-linking reagent SPDP. The monoclonal antibody-C3b conjugate promoted the killing of K562 tumor cells by normal human serum. Treatment of the tumor cells with the monoclonal antibody and normal human serum resulted in 10-15% lysis. However, following pretreatment of the cells with antibody-C3b conjugates, their lysis by normal human serum increased to 70%. The conjugate activated selectively the alternative pathway of complement and the C3b component in the conjugate was highly resistant to cleavage and inactivation by the complement regulatory proteins Factors H and I. These results suggest that the coupling of C3b molecules to monoclonal antibodies anti-unique tumor antigens produces a potent complement-activating reagent which may act specifically on tumor cells and promote cancer therapy.

REFERENCES

1. Müller-Eberhard, H. J., and Schreiber, R. D. (1980). Molecular biology and chemistry of the alternative pathway of complement. *Adv. Immunol. 29*: 1-53.
2. Müller-Eberhard, H. J., and Götze, O. (1972). C3 proactivator convertase and its mode of action. *J. Exp. Med. 135*:1003-1008.
3. Fearon, D. T., Austen, K. F., and Ruddy, S. (1973). Formation of a hemolytically active cellular intermediate by the interaction between properdin Factors B and D and the activated third component of complement. *J. Exp. Med. 138*:1305-1313.
4. Fishelson, Z., Pangburn, M. K., and Müller-Eberhard, H. J. (1983). C3 convertase of the alternative complement pathway. Demonstration of an active, stable C3b,Bb(Ni) complex. *J. Biol. Chem. 258*:7411-7415.
5. Müller-Eberhard, H. J. (1986). The membrane attack complement of complement. *Ann. Rev. Immunol. 4*:503-528.
6. Pangburn, M. K., and Müller-Eberhard, H. J. (1978). Complement C3 convertase: Cell surface restriction of β1H control and generation of restriction in neuraminidase treated cells. *Proc. Natl. Acad. Sci. USA 75*:2416-2420.

7. Weiler, J. M., Daha, M. R., Austen, K. F., and Fearon, D. T. (1976). Control of the amplification convertase of complement by the plasma protein β1H. *Proc. Natl. Acad. Sci. USA 73*:3268–3272.

8. Gaither, T. A., Hammer, C. H., and Frank, M. M. (1979). Studies of the molecular mechanisms of C3b inactivation and a simplified assay of β1H and the C3b inactivator (C3b INA). *J. Immunol. 123*:1195–1204.

9. Pangburn, M. K., Schreiber, R. D., and Müller-Eberhard, H. J. (1977). Human complement C3b inactivator: Isolation, characterization and demonstration of an absolute requirement for the serum protein β1H for cleavage of C3b and C4b in solution. *J. Exp. Med. 146*:257–270.

10. Law, S. K., Fearon, D. T., and Levine, R. P. (1979). Action of the C3b-inactivator on cell-bound C3b. *J. Immunol. 122*:759–765.

11. Mayer, M. M. (1961). Development of the one-hit theory of immune hemolysis. *Immunochemical Approaches to Problems in Microbiology*. Edited by M. Heidelberger and O. J. Plescia. Rutgers University Press, New Brunswick, NJ, pp. 268–279.

12. Koski, C. L., Ramm, L. E., Hammer, C. H., Mayer, M. M., and Shin, M. L. (1983). Cytolysis of nucleated cells by complement: cell death displays multi-hit characteristics. *Proc. Natl. Acad. Sci. USA 80*:3816–3820.

13. Nicholson-Weller, A., Burge, J., Fearon, D. T., Weller, P. F., and Austen, K. F. (1982). Isolation of a human erythrocyte membrane glycoprotein with decay-accelerating activity for C3 convertase of the complement system. *J. Immunol. 129*:184–189.

14. Fearon, D. T. (1979). Regulation of the amplification C3 convertase of human complement by an inhibitory protein isolated from human erythrocyte membrane. *Proc. Natl. Acad. Sci. USA 76*:5867–5871.

15. Zalman, L. S., Wood, L. M., and Müller-Eberhard, H. J. (1986). Isolation of a human erythrocyte membrane protein capable of inhibiting expression of homologous complement transmembrane channels. *Proc. Natl. Acad. Sci. USA 83*:6975–6979.

16. Ohanian, S. H., and Schlager, S. I. (1981). Humoral immune killing of nucleated cells: Mechanisms of complement-mediated attack and target cell defense. *CRC Crit. Rev. Immunol. 1*:165–209.

17. Köhler, G., and Milstein, C. (1975). Continuous cultures of fused cells secreting antibody of predefined specificity. *Nature (Lond.) 256*:495–497.

18. Vitetta, E. S., and Uhr, J. W. (1985). Immunotoxins. *Ann. Rev. Immunol. 3*:197–212.

19. Vogel, C. W., and Müller-Eberhard, H. J. (1981). Induction of immune cytolysis: Tumor-cell killing by complement is initiated by covalent complex of monoclonal antibody and stable C3/C5 convertase. *Proc. Natl. Acad. Sci. USA 78*:7707–7711.

20. Parker, C. J., White, V. F., and Falk, R. J. (1986). Site-specific activation of the alternative pathway of complement. Synthesis of a hybrid molecule consisting of antibody and cobra venom factor. *Complement 3*:223–235.

21. Newman, R., Schneider, C., Sutherland, R., Vodinelick, L., and Greaves, M. (1982). The transferrin receptor. *Trends. Biochem. Sci. 1*:397–400.

22. Gatter, K. C., Brown, G., Trowbridge, I., Woolston, R. E., and Mason, D. Y. (1983). Transferrin receptor in human tissues: their distribution and possible clinical relevance. *J. Clin. Pathol. 36*:539–545.

23. Hammer, C. H., Wirtz, G. H., Renfer, L., Gersham, H. D., and Tack, B. F. (1981). Large scale isolation of functionally active components of the human complement system. *J. Biol. Chem. 256*:3995–4006.

24. Isenman, D. E., Kells, D. I. C., Cooper, N. R., Müller-Eberhard, H. J., and Pangburn, M. K. (1981). Nucleophilic modification of human complement protein C3: Correlation of conformational changes with acquisition of C3b-like functional properties. *Biochemistry 20*:4458–4467.

25. Fraker, P. J., and Speck, J. C., Jr. (1978). Protein and cell membrane iodination with a sparingly soluble chloramide 1,3,4,6-tetrachloro-3a,6a-diphenylglycoluril. *Biochem. Biophys. Res. Comm. 80*:849–857.

26. Lozzio, B. B., and Lozzio, C. B. (1979). Properties and usefulness of the original K 562 human myelogenous leukemia cell line. *Leukemia Res. 3*: 363–370.

27. Carrlsson, J., Drevin, H., and Axen, R. (1978). Protein thiolation and reversible protein-protein conjugation, N-succinimidyl 3-(2-pyridyldithio)-propionate, a new heterobifunctional reagent. *Biochem. J. 173*:723–737.

28. Laemmli, U. K. (1970). Cleavage of structural proteins during the assembly of the head of bacteriophage T4. *Nature (Lond.) 227*:680–685.

29. Shin, M. L., Hänsch, G., Hu, V. W., and Nicholson-Weller, A. (1986). Membrane factors responsible for homologous species restriction of complement-mediated lysis: Evidence for a factor other than DAF operating at the stage of C8 and C9. *J. Immunol. 136*:1777–1782.

30. Des Prez, R. M., Bryan, C. S., Hawiger, J., and Colley, D. G. (1975). Function of the classical and alternate pathways of human complement in serum treated with ethylene glycol tetraacetic acid and $MgCl_2$-ethylene glycol tetraacetic acid. *Infect. Immun. 11*:1235–1243.

31. Fishelson, Z. and Reiter, Y. Monoclonal antibody–C3b conjugates: Killing of K562 cells and selection of a stable complement resistant variant. *Mechanisms of Action and Therapeutic Application of Biologicals in Cancer and Immune Deficiency Disorders*. Edited by J. Groopman, C. Evans, and D. Golde. Allan R. Liss Inc., New York, NY (in press).

32. Fishelson, Z. (1985). Cell triggering by activated complement components. *Immunol. Lett. 11*:261–276.

33. Ross, G. D., and Medof, M. E. (1985). Membrane complement receptors specific for bound fragments of C3. *Adv. Immunol. 37*:217–267.

7

Marrow Purging for Autologous Bone Marrow Transplantation

VALÉRIE COMBARET, M. C. FAVROT, AND T. PHILIP
Centre Léon Berard, Lyon, France

I. INTRODUCTION

In the management of leukemia and malignant solid tumors (if one excepts the graft versus leukemia (GVL) effect of an allograft), allogenic or autologous bone marrow transplantations (BMT) are not therapeutic per se, but simply method-designed to overcome myelotoxicity after high-dose chemotherapy. The main limitations of this method are presentation of graft versus host disease (GVHD) in allogenic BMT, and the contamination of the graft by residual malignant cells in autologous BM. A common approach, so called "purging," has been proposed to eliminate unwanted cells, either allogenic normal T cells responsible for GVHD or autologous malignant cells, from the BM before its reinjection. This "ex vivo manipulation" represents only one step of a complete process that includes high-dose chemotherapy and BMT. The interest of the "purging procedures," especially for autografting, is then strictly linked to the future of high-dose chemotherapy and the attitude is controversial, depending on the disease: in solid tumors or leukemia, and in terms of timing and efficiency of the high-dose chemotherapy during the course of the disease. It is already clear that indications could be widened and patients grafted at very early stages of the disease; in such indications, very sensitive methods are required to determine whether the BM is free from disease, especially in cases of leukemia, and for this reason requires no purging. It still remains to be proved whether results of high-dose chemotherapy and BMT would be better than those of conventional therapy and whether the potential toxicity of the whole procedure could be reduced to acceptably low levels. On the contrary, indications of BM autografting, especially in cases of solid tumors, could be restricted to high-risk patients in partial remission, relapse or even progression; our view is that the purging is likely to be necessary in most cases, but the clinical relevance and efficacy of such a procedure might only be demonstrated when the residual disease outside the bone marrow is totally eliminated by high-dose chemotherapy. The final attitude could be to harvest the BM early in the course of the disease but to reserve BMT for relapsing patients; even if theoretically ideal and feasible in few patients, it will not be applicable on a large scale in solid tumors because of considerations of cost and availability of resources, but it is worthy of consideration in leukemia.

II. PURGING TECHNOLOGY

One usually distinguishes between physical, chemical, and immunological methods.

A. Physical Separation

These techniques, such as Percoll or bovine serum albumin gradient, were the first methods described (1), and more recently, techniques such as counterflow centrifugation have been published (2). The selection of hematopoietic precursors for reinfusion is based on their density. These methods are not as efficient as recent procedures but can be used as a preliminary step for a more effective separation (2). Soybean lectin separation has been shown to allow a poor elimination of neuroblastoma cells or T- and B-cell acute lymphoblastic leukemia (B-ALL) cells (3).

B. Chemical Methods

These consist of applying chemotherapeutic agents which may destroy malignant cells with at least a partial preservation of normal hematopoietic progenitors (4,5). Although this last point is still very unclear (6), active derivatives of cyclophosphamide, either 4-HC (4-hydroxycyclophosphamide) or ASTA Z 7557 (mafosfamid), are now extensively used in clinical trials, especially for autografting in ALL or acute myeloid leukemia (AML) (7–11). This drug has been tested experimentally or used in clinics for solid tumors such as non-Hodgkin malignant lymphoma (NHML) (11) or neuroblastoma (12). The clinical use of other chemotherapeutic agents, such as etoposide (13), single or in association (14), has not yet been started on a large scale. Some nonchemotherapeutic agents have potential interest, such as merocyamine 540, a DNA dye with lytic activity after photoactivation (15), or 6-OH dopamine with selective toxicity on neuroblastoma cells (16).

C. Immunological Methods

These methods allow unwanted cells to be specifically targeted by monoclonal antibodies (MAbs) directed against cell surface antigens. These cells are then eliminated by various mechanisms.

1. Complement-Dependent Lysis

MAbs (IgM or IgG_2a isotypes) lyse targeted cells in the presence of rabbit complement (17–21). Some of these MAbs, such as AL_2 and mouse MAbs $RFAL_3$, RFB_7, BA_1, BA_2, and BA_3 are claimed to be lytic against leukemic cells in the presence of human complement (22,23) as well as BG_6 lytic against neuroblastoma cells (24).

2. Immunomagnetic Depletion

Magnetic particles (either macro particles or colloids) covered with anti-mouse immunoglobulins attach malignant cells covered with specific MoAbs through a linkage between the anti-mouse immunoglobulins and the MAbs and the coated cells are removed by a magnetic field (25–29). A few other methods derive from the same principle: for example malignant cells can be absorbed in a column via the reaction between avidin- and biotin-labeled antibodies (30).

3. Immunotoxins

MAbs are conjugated to toxins. Ricin is the most commonly studied and used in clinical trials (31). This consists of two chains: the toxic A chain acts inside the cell by inhibiting protein synthesis on the 60S subunit of ribosomes; the B chain acts at the surface like a monovalent lectin, binding to galactose and N-galactosamine residues on the cell, and attaches the toxin to the membrane. The lytic activity of the ricin A chain is long (1 or 2 days) and is influenced by the presence or absence of the B chain, the affinity of the MAbs, the temperature, and the pH of incubation (32–35). In spite of these disadvantages, immunotoxins are probably the most efficient drugs which act in the presence of NH_4Cl_2 at very low concentrations. Toxins or activators with potential clinical interest are coupled either on MAbs directed against B-cell or T-cell leukemic blasts or MAbs directed against solid tumors (36–40).

Table 1 Purging Methods for Autologous Bone Marrow Transplantation: Experimental and Clinical Assays [footnotes on p. 142]

| | | Experimental Assays | |
| | | Method of quantification[a] | (limit of detection) |
Methods	Model		
Complement-dependent lysis			
MoAbs			
J_5 (CD$_{10}$)	C-ALL	^{51}Cr (BM + 1% tumor cells or 1% Nalm1)	(2 log)
BA$_1$ (CD$_{24}$)	C-ALL	Clon. assay	(>4 log)
BA$_2$ (CD$_9$)	pre-B ALL	(BM + 5% KM$_3$, HPB-null	
BA$_3$ (CD$_{10}$)		Nalm6)	
J_5 (CD$_{10}$)	BL	Clon. assay	(>5 log)
J_2 (CD$_9$)		(BM + 1% MANALWA)	
B$_1$ (CD$_{20}$)			
B$_1$ (CD$_{20}$)	BL	Liquid culture ass.	(4–5 log)
Y29/55		(BM + 1% Daudi, Raji, LY$_{67}$	
AL$_2$ (CD$_{10}$)		IARC BL$_{17}$, BL$_{63}$, BL$_{93}$ or tumor cells)	
Y29/55	B-CLL	IF (tumor cells)	(2.5 log)
RFAL $_3$ or CD$_7$ (+ second Ab when required)	C-ALL T-ALL	TdT assay on tumor cells	(>4 log)
Immunomagnetic depletion			
MoABs			
UJ13A, UJ223.8	Neuroblastoma	Immunofluoresence	(?)
UJ127.11,		Clonogenic assay	
UJ181.4		(BM + 1% CHP100)	
Thy-1, H11			
Thy-1, H11	Neuroblastoma	Physical parameters defined on BL model (see text)	(5 log)
Ab390, Ab459,	Neuroblastoma	Hoescht 342	(4 log)
HSAN 1.2		(BM + 20% LAN-1)	
BA$_1$, RFB$_{21.7}$		SHS-KCNR	
(± BA$_2$, leu 7)		SH-S KANR	
		LA-N-5	
Chemical methods: 4HC or mafosfamid			
4-HC or	AML	Rat model (LCFU-S)	
mafosfamid	AML	Clonogenic assay 100% tumor cells	(?)
	AML	Clonogenic assay BM + 5% tumor cells	(?)
	ALL	Clonogenic assay BM + cell lines	(8 log)
	ALL		
	ALL		
	ALL		

	Clinical Assays			
			Toxicity[b] (median-days)	
Elimination	Patients (n)	Neutrophils	Platelets	Reference(s)
99%	24	44 (16–78)	50 (16–103)	(19,65)
2–4 log	23	22 (16–64)	34 (7–78)	(22,66)
1–3.5 log	8 (LMNH)[c]	30 (14–57)	28 (18–60)	(20,67)
1–4 log	12	17 (5–22)	33 (13–56)	(21,47,55)
2.5 log	7 (BL)[c]	14 (10–36)	27 (8–117)	(68,69)
4 log	18	24 (15–66)	36 (24–140)	(50,19)
99.9%	17	22 (14–36)	33 (14–43)	(25,26)
	4 (grafted after relapse)	46	81.5	
4–5 log on BL model	44	24	39	(70) (26,27)
3–4 log	14	?	?	(28,71)
5–6 log	25	29 (16–63)	57 (23–191)	(4,7)
?	14	34 (19–47)	150 (55–330)	(8,72)
	16	27 (14–50)	45 (13–90)	(9)
Lack of specific reactivity for malignant cells				(5)
6 log				(38)
	21	25 (13–60)	33 (14–33)	(11)
	5	(15–28)	(23–35)	(10)
	8	19 (11–30)	50 (23–90)	(8)

III. BM PURGING PROCEDURES FOR
AUTOLOGOUS BMT (Table 1)

In the standardization of purging methods for autologous BMT, two different
aspects have to be considered: the technology itself and a model for testing its
efficiency, with a clear distinction between experimental models and clinical
assessment. The potentially optimal method may vary from one disease to
another, depending upon the features of the malignant cells studied; the efficiency is different when the method is used on cell lines or on fresh tumor
samples. In a few clinical situations of autografting, malignant cells can effectively be detected in the graft, warranting the efforts made to remove such cells;
the logical criteria for using such purging methods in practice are that the
efficiency and the lack of toxicity for hematopoietic precursors have already
been well proven experimentally and that the method applied in clinical practice
is reproducible and efficient on large numbers of BM cells. Rigorous methods to
detect and eliminate malignant cells will then be necessary to justify the routine
application of the purging methods and consider the possibility of any extensive
or even randomized multicentric study.

A. Experimental Models

Experimental models on animals have been initiated, suggesting that purging
methods can eliminate leukemic cells from an autograft (leukemic cells have
been the most extensively investigated) and have predicted the feasibility of
autologous BMT (41–43). However, none of the animal models studied to date
provides a precise analogue for autologous BMT in humans and syngeneic tumor
transplants have been studied rather than primary autochthonous tumors. The
capacity of various methods to purge a 100% malignant population has been
demonstrated using the ^{51}Cr release assay, the measure of thymidine incorporation or [^{125}I] UDR (uridine deoxyribo) uptake (44). More recently, efforts
have been made to demonstrate the efficiency of the purging methods in models

---

Table 1 (continued)

[a]Experiments were performed on either 100% cells, or on a mixture of irradiated marrow
and malignant cells; "tumors" refer to noncultured malignant cells; cell lines are entered
under reference name. ^{51}Cr = measure of the ^{51}Cr-release, clon. ass. = clonogenic assay
with limited dilutions.
[b]Toxicity: number of days necessary to obtain 0.5×10^9 neutrophils/liter or 50×10^9
platelets/liter.
[c]When the experimental model and the clinical model are different, the disease is defined
between parentheses.

closer to the clinical situation, namely bone marrow samples contaminated with 1 to 10% malignant cells from various malignant cell lines. Either semisolid or liquid culture assays allowed to quantify up to 6 log elimination, using limited dilutions and pre-B, T, null, or common ALL cell lines, or Burkitt lymphoma (BL) cell lines (17,20,45). However, there are limitations to such systems, the main one being the use of very selected cell lines known to have a high clonogenic efficiency. Such models did not therefore allow to demonstrate variations due to the heterogeneity of the tumor samples. An interesting alternative method for the detection of residual malignant cells has been described when cell lines such as those established from solid tumors have a very low clonogenic efficiency. The staining of cell lines by vital dye Hoescht 342 before their admixture with the BM allows a further objective and rapid detection of as few as 1 in 10^4 malignant cells by a visual analysis. Reynolds et al. (46) published the detection of as few as 10^{-6} residual malignant cells by a computerized analysis; however, this method can only measure an immediate elimination of cells (i.e., complement lysis or immunomagnetic depletion) but is inappropriate to test the related lytic activity of drugs; it is again restricted to artificial models of BM contaminated with cell lines.

B. Clinical or Preclinical Assessment of the Purging Methods

In opposition with previous experimental models, some methods of detection allow to assay the purging method both on bone marrow artificially contaminated with cultured malignant cells and on marrow samples freshly obtained from patients. Again, these methods can be divided into two groups, depending on the proliferative potential of malignant cells. We recently developed a liquid cell culture assay, though restricted to the Burkitt lymphoma model, which enabled us to detect one residual malignant cell in 10^6 normal BM cells in short-term culture (10 days), and to detect a single residual BL cell in the BM sample in long-term culture (21 days). The BM can be contaminated with Epstein-Barr virus negative or positive (EBV) cell lines recently established from our patients who are candidates for an autograft, or even with their own noncultured tumor cells from the primary tumor (47). Such an assay allows quantification in experimental or in clinical assays, of up to 5 log elimination of malignant cells from BM contaminated with 1% BL cells. Other published assays usually quantify the purging efficiency on populations of 100% tumor cells. Ajani et al. (48) describe a human solid tumor stem cell assay to test the efficiency of drugs (clonogenic efficiency = 1%) and Uckun et al. (49) a colony assay to evaluate the cytotoxicity of immunotoxins on common B-ALL (clonogenic efficiency = 0.09–2.63%). Because the clonogenic efficiency of such tumor samples is very low, other groups developed methods based on immunostaining or dye exclusion.

Campana and Janossy (50) showed that double staining with TdT and a specific membrane marker allows detection of greater than 4 log elimination of acute common pre-B or pre-T lymphoblastic leukemic cells. BuDR incorporation by malignant cells proves that such cell populations are really the proliferating malignant cells. Similarly and as described by others (51), we showed that 10^{-4} to 10^{-5} residual neuroblastoma cells can be detected in the BM by an immunocytochemical staining. Finally, Laurent et al. (52) described a semiquantitative dye exclusion assay to test routinely the sensitivity of either T-ALL or B-CLL to T_{101} immunotoxin (FOA staining of living cells and PI staining of dead cells). Any of these assays allows a relatively quick and reproducible evaluation of the potential efficiency of any purging procedure for an individual patient.

Even more important with regard to the whole concept of the reinjection of a purged autograft, immunostaining methods or culture assays (if the clonogenic efficiency is sufficient, as in our BL model) allows ascertainment of whether or not the BM contains residual malignant cells (as few as 10^{-4} to 10^{-5}) when harvested, and to demonstrate their elimination by the purging methods. It is indeed fundamental, if one wants to evaluate the efficacy of any purging method for autografting, to clearly distinguish published reports of patients grafted in relapse or partial remission with BM involvement, but who received an autograft taken in first complete remission (CR) from the rare reports of patients harvested and grafted in partial remission (PR) or relapse with residual malignant cells in the BM before the purging procedure. For example, in none of our Stage IV BL cases does the BM contain BL cells detectable by the liquid cell culture assay when the patients achieve first CR and, consequently, if harvested at such period, the BM would probably not need purging. On the other hand, in 40% patients in relapse the cytologically normal BM dose contain growing BL cells; in 2 of our 30 patients harvested and grafted either in PR or second CR, the harvested BM contained BL cells detected only by the liquid cell culture assay before the purging procedure and eliminated after the purging (53,54). Similarly, Janossy et al. demonstrated, in 2 ALL patients transplanted in relapse, a contamination of the BM by TdT + blast cells before the purging procedure and their disappearance to levels undetectable by the TdT assay (18,50). In our group of 45 unselected patients with Stage IV neuroblastoma entered in the autograft program, 13 had a pathological BM when harvested, but in 9 of them, malignant cells were detectable only in the trephine biopsies, whereas in 4 others clumps of neuroblasts were detectable by immunocytology in the harvested BM before purging (55). Similar neuroblastoma cases with malignant cells in the harvested BM were reported by Kemshead et al. (56). The case histories of these patients who had pathological BM at the time of harvesting and grafting and who further achieved a BM CR under high-dose chemotherapy supports the rationale of the purging procedure in such a therapeutic approach. Indeed, the patients will receive at least 10^4 malignant cells/kg unless purging is performed;

even if the percentage of malignant cells which can find an appropriate micro-
environment for regenerating the malignant clone once they were reinjected
into the patient, is unknown, it is difficult to consider that none of these are
clonogenic after reinjection.

C. Comparison of the "Purging" Methods and Their Combinations

In the BL model, De Fabriitis et al. (57) demonstrated 2 to 3.5 log elimination
of clonogenic cells in five different cell lines,either by a complement-dependent
lysis procedure (with 3 MAbs, $J_5 + J_2 + B_1$) or 4-HC. The combination of both
methods slightly improved the BM cleansing. Lebien et al. (58) similarly showed
either an improvement of the malignant cell elimination by combining mafosfamid and a complement lysis procedure (with $BA_1 + BA_2 + BA_3$) on B-ALL cell
lines, or some complementary effects when the lines were resistant to one or the
other procedure. Finally, Uckun et al. (37) showed 7 to 8 log elimination of
target B-ALL cell lines by a combination of mafosfamid and a B-cell-directed
immunotoxin (B43-PAP). The main conclusion of these three authors is a variation observed among samples. This is probably accentuated by the difference of
proliferative capacity. In these systems, the ASTA.Z 7557 activity might be
overestimated as target cells that were used are rapidly dividing cell lines, different from some resting leukemic cell population.

We recently compared the efficiency of two different immunological proced
ures, the complement lysis and the immunomagnetic depletion (IMD) in the BL
model (Table 2). We previously demonstrated that three MAbs (B_1, Y29/55, and
AL_2) are capable of 3 to 4 log BL-cell elimination with complement lysis (21).
The lytic activity of a cocktail of two MAbs (SB_4 and RFB_7) showed an even
better lysis in all experiments. With B_1 as a single MAb, the IMD allows a 4 to 5 log
depletion, using a mononuclear BM cell fraction rather than buffy coat and a
double-depletion procedure (26,27). The BL_{99} and BL_2 cell lines were very
sensitive to the complement lysis, and in contrast, the BL_{93} cell line was partially resistant to the complement lysis, irrespective of the MAb cocktail selected. In the case of BL_{93}, an optimal BL cell elimination was achieved with the
immunomagnetic method. It appears therefore that the two immunological
procedures are complementary (Table 3) (59). The different qualities of MAbs
required (i.e., IgM for complement lysis and IgG for magnetic beads) could explain the results. Whereas some MAbs, such as SB_4, are highly cytotoxic with
rabbit complement, even when the antigen they react with is weakly expressed,
the immunomagnetic procedure requires MAbs of high affinity and high density
on cells. Preliminary experiments even suggest that the use of MAb cocktails
does not necessarily improve the efficiency of immunomagnetic depletion,
but may even decrease its depleting power (27).

Table 2 Comparison of Two Immunological Purging Procedures

	Complement-dependent lysis procedure		
	$RFB_7 + SB_4$	$B_1 + AL_2$ + Y29/55	Immunomagnetic depletion
BL_{99} n = 8 EBV + (8,22) Caucasian	5	5	4
BL_{93} n = 5 EBV(−) (8,14) Caucasian	3	2.5	5
BL_2 n = 5 EBV(−) (8,22) Caucasian	5	5	4

The efficiency of the procedure has been evaluated by the liquid cell culture assay in short- and long-term culture and results are expressed in decimal logarithms (means of 5 to 8 experiments) (when BL cell growth was fully inhibited and all BL cells then eliminated from the sample, cytoreduction was recorded as 5 log). Experiments with complement lysis and IMD were performed on the same samples and on the same day. Irradiated normal BM samples were contaminated with 1% BL cells from three different cell lines recently established from our patients.

Table 3 Complementary Effects of Two Immunological Procedures

	Complement	Magnetic Depletion
BL_{99}	5	2
BL_{93}	2	5
BL_2	5	3

These three individual experiments (1 on each line) are part of Table 2 results and given as examples: when one of the two techniques fails, the other one is highly efficient.
Results are expressed in logarithms.

As suggested by various groups, it is tempting to combine these methods; we will not, however, advocate doing so. Indeed, the fact that some of the purging methods described above are capable, when combined, of removing large quantities of malignant cells is only of theoretical interest. The BM contamination reflects a resistance of malignant cells to chemotherapy, and if such contamination is important, the residual disease outside the BM is likely to be resistant to high-dose chemotherapy. The most successful clinical application of purging is therefore likely to be on BM harvested from patients within minimal involvement (i.e., 1% or less malignant cells). The only interest in combining procedures will thus be to overcome, for a few patients, the possible resistance of malignant cells to one or the other procedure. However such an attitude will lead, for all other patients, to a higher toxicity and practical difficulties. An option might be to select the most effective MAbs, or even the most suitable procedure, to be used on malignant tumor samples from each individual patient, with relatively quick and reproducible assays such as those described above. The definition of the efficiency of the purging procedure for these patients will help further clinical analysis.

IV. CONCLUSION

Results recently published by Saarinen et al. (24) on the autograft of AML patients in relapse (or subsequent complete remission) already provide evidence that the 4-OH purging procedure, shown to be efficient experimentally, may have a beneficial effect in this disease. However, in most clinical models, the evidence of purging efficacy is difficult to prove on the basis of analysis of clinical results. When relapse does occur, it is impossible to ascertain whether it is due to residual disease resistant to chemotherapy or to disease reinjected with the BM. Until recently, in most clinical trials, there was no proof that the BM was infiltrated by tumor and thus needed to be purged, and also no method for demonstrating total freedom from tumor. Partial answers have to be initially obtained in clinical models, using rigorously controlled purging procedures together with methods sensitive enough to detect a minimal number of residual malignant cells in the BM.Such a rigorous analysis of the clinical value of purging methods is fundamental to future prospects, as well as the survey of the role of high-dose chemotherapy andABMT in the management of malignant proliferations. Selective in vitro maintenance of normal hematopoietic progenitors (60) or the positive selection of such progenitors with relevant MAbs (61) could be an alternative to the reinjection of the whole BM mononuclear cell fraction after purging. Transplantation with peripheral blood hematopoietic cells could be another alternative if the lack of circulating malignant cells, when the BM is involved, is clearly demonstrated (62,63). Even further therapeutic approaches, such as in vitro immunostimulation of the patient's effector cells, will involve ex vivo manipulation of either peripheral or BM mononuclear cells (64). The autografting technology developed in the last decade then appears to be a preliminary but essential step for the introduction of new immunological developments in therapy.

REFERENCES

1. Dicke, K. A., Zander, A., Spitzer, G., Verma, D. S., Peters, L., Vellekoop, L., and McCredie, K. B. (1979). Autologous bone marrow transplantation in adult acute leukemia in relapse. *Lancet 1*:514.
2. Figdor, C. G., Voute, P. A., De Kraker, J., Vernier, L. N., and Bont, W. S. (1985). Physical cell separation of neuroblastoma cells from bone marrow. *Adv. Neuroblast. Res. 175*:459.
3. Reisner, Y. (1983). Differential agglutination by soybean agglutinin of human leukemia and neuroblastoma cell lines: potential application to autologous bone marrow transplantation. *Proc. Natl. Acad. Sci. USA 80*:6657.
4. Kaizer, H., Cote, J. P., and Sharkis, S. (1982). Autologous bone marrow transplantation in acute leukemia: the use of in vitro incubation of tumor-marrow mixtures with 4-hydroxyperoxycyclophosphamide (4 HC) in a Wistar-Furth rat model of acute myelogenous leukemia (WF-AML). *Proc. Assoc. Cancer Res. 23*:194.
5. Korbling, M., Hess, A. D., Tutschka, P. J., Kaiser, H., Colvin, M. O., and Santos, G. W. (1982). 4-Hydroxyperoxycyclophosphamide: a model for eliminating residual human tumour cells and T-lymphocytes from the bone marrow graft. *Br. J. Haematol. 52*:89.
6. Kluin-Nelemans, H. C., Martens, A. C. M., Lowenberg, B., and Hagenbeek, A. (1984). No preferential sensitivity of clonogenic AML cells to Asta Z 7557. *Leukemia Res. 8*:723.
7. Yeager, A. M., Kaizer, J., Santos, G. W., Saral, R., Colvin, O. M., Stuart, R. K., Braine, H. G., Burke, P. J., Ambinder, R. F., and Burns, W. H. (1986). Autologous bone marrow transplantation in patient with acute non-lymphocytic leukemia, using ex vivo marrow treatment with 4-hydroxyperoxycyclophosphamide. *N. Engl. J. Med. 315*:141.
8. Gorin, N. C., Douay, L., Laporte, J. P., Lopez, M., Mary, J. Y., Najman, A., Salmon, C., Aagerter, P., Stachowiak, J., David, R., Pene, F., Kantor, G., Deloux, J., Duhamel, E., Van den Akker, J., Gerota, J., Parlier, Y., and Duhamel, G. (1986). Autologous bone marrow transplantation using marrow incubated with Asta Z 7557 in adult acute leukemia. *Blood 67*:1367.
9. Cahn, J. Y., Hervé, P., Flesch, M., Plouvier, E., Noir, A., Racadot, E., Montcuquet, P., Benar, C., Pignon, B., Boilletot, A., Lutz, P., Henon, P., Rozenbaum, A., Peters, A., and Leconte des Floris, R. (1986). Autologous bone marrow transplantation (ABMT) for acute leukaemia in complete remission: a pilot study on 33 cases. *Br. J. Haematol. 63*:457

10. Hervé, P., Cahn, J. Y., Plouvier, E., Fleshc, M., Tamayo, E., Leconte des Floris, R., and Peters, A. (1984). Autologous bone marrow transplantation for acute leukemia using transplant chemopurified with metabolite of oxazaphosphorines (ASTA Z 7557), INN mafosfamide). First clinical results. *New Drugs 2*:245.

11. Kaizer, H., Stuart, R. K., Brookmeyer, R., Beschorner, W. E., Braine, H. G., Burns, W. H., Fuller, D. J., Korbling, M., Mangan, K. F., Saral, R., Sensenbrenner, L., Shadduck, R. K., Shende, A. C., Tutschka, P. J., Yeager, A. M., Zinkham, W. H., Colvin, O. M., and Santos, G. W. (1985). Autologous bone marrow transplantation in acute leukemia: a phase I study of in vitro treatment of marrow with 4-hydroxyperoxycyclophosphamide to purge tumor cells. *Blood 65*:1504.

12. Hartmann, O., Kalifa, C., Beaujean, F., Bayle, C., Benhamou, E., Lemerle, J. Treatment of advanced neuroblastoma with two consecutive high-dose chemotherapy regimens and ABMT. *Adv. Neuroblast. Res. 175*:565-568.

13. Ciobanu, N., Paietta, E., Andreeff, M., Papenhausen, P., and Wiernik, P. H. (1986). Etoposide as an in vitro purging agent for the treatment of acute leukemias and lymphomas in conjunction with autologous bone marrow transplantation. *Exp. Hematol. 14*:626.

14. Chang, T. T., Gulati, S. C., Chou, T. C., Vega, R., Gandola, L., Ezzat Ibrahim, S. M., Yopp, J., Colvin, M., and Clarkson, B. D. (1985). Synergistic effect of 4-hydroxyperoxycyclophosphamide and etoposide on a human promyelocytic leukemia cell line (HL-60) demonstrated by computer analysis. *Cancer Res. 45*:2434.

15. Sieber, F., Spivak, J. L., and Sutcliffe, A. M. (1984). Selective killing of leukemic cells by perocyanine 540-mediated photosensitization. *Proc. Natl. Acad. Sci. USA 81*:7584.

16. Reynolds, C. P., Reynolds, D. A., Frenkel, E. P., and Graham Smith, R. (1982). Selective toxicity of 6-hydroxydopamine and ascorbate for human neuroblastoma in vitro: amodel for clearing marrow prior to autologous transplant. *Cancer Res. 42*:1331.

17. Lebien, T. W., Stepan, D. E., Bartholomew, R. M., Stong, R. C., and Anderson, J. M. (1985). Utilization of a colony assay to assess the variables influencing elimination of leukemic cells from human bone marrow with monoclonal antibodies and complement. *Blood 65*:945.

18. Janossy, G., Campana, D., Galton, J., Burnett, A., Hann, I., Grob, J. P., Prentice, H. G., and Totterman, T. (1986). Applications of monoclonal antibodies in bone marrow transplantation (BMT). *3rd Workshop on Leucocyte Differentiation Antigens*. Oxford, New York. (in press).

19. Bast, R. C., Ritz, J., Lipton, J. M., Feeney, M., Sallan, S. E., Nathan, D. G., and Schlossman, S. F. (1983). Elimination of leukemic cells from human bone marrow using monoclonal antibody and complement. *Cancer Res. 43*:1389.

20. Bast, R. C., De Fabriitis, P., Lipton, J., Gelber, R., Maver, C., Nadler, L., Sallan, S., and Ritz, J. (1985). Elimination of malignant clonogenic cells from human bone marrow using multiple monoclonal antibodies and complement. *Cancer Res. 45*:499.

21. Favrot, M. C., Philip, L., Philip, T., Pinkerton, R., Lebacq, A. M., Forster, K., Adeline, P., and Doré, J. F. (1986). Bone marrow purging procedure in Burkitt lymphoma with monoclonal antibodies and complement. Quantification by a liquid cell culture monitoring system. *Br. J. Cancer 64*:161.
22. Stepan, D. E., Bartholomew, R. M., and Lebien, T. W. (1984). In vitro cytodestruction of human leukemic cells using murine monoclonal antibodies and human complement. *Blood 63*:1120.
23. Lebacq-Verheyden, A. M., Humblet, Y., Ravoet, A. M., and Symann, M. (1984). Immunological removal of cancer cells in bone marrow autografts: setting the experimental conditions. *Autologous Bone Marrow Transplantation in Solid Tumors*. Edited by J. G. McVie, O. Dalesio, and I. E. Smith. Raven Press, New York, pp. 19–28.
24. Saarinen, M., Coccia, P. F., Gerson, S. L., Pelley, R., and Cheung, N. K. V. (1985). Eradication of neuroblastoma cells in vitro by monoclonal antibody and human complement: method for purging autologous bone marrow. *Cancer Res. 45*:5969.
25. Treleaven, J. G., Gibson, F. M., Ugelstad, J., Rembaum, A., Philip, T., Caine, G. D., and Kemshead, J. T. (1984). Removal of neuroblastoma cells from bone marrow with monoclonal antibodies conjugated to magnetic micropheres. *Lancet 14*:70.
26. Favrot, M. C., Philip, I., Combaret, V., Maritaz, O., and Philip, T. (1987). Experimental evaluation of an immunomagnetic bone marrow purging procedure using the Burkitt lymphoma model. *Bone Marrow Trans. 2*:59–66.
27. Combaret, V., Favrot, M. C., Kremens, B., Laurent, J. C., Philip, I., and Philip, T. (1986). Elimination of Burkitt cells from excess bone marrow with an immunomagnetic purging procedure. Selection of monoclonal antibodies is a critical step. *Proceedings of the Second International Symposium on ABMT*, Houston, In press.
28. Reynolds, P. C., Seeger, R. C., Vo, D. D., Black, A. T., Wells, J., and Ugelstad, J. (1986). Model system for removing neuroblastoma cells from bone marrow using monoclonal antibodies and magnetic immunobeads. *Cancer Res. 46*:5882.
29. Poynton, C. H., Dicke, K. A., Culbert, S., Frankel, L. S., Jagannath, S., and Reading, C. L. (1983). Immunomagnetic removal of CALLA positive cells from human bone marrow. *Lancet i*:524.
30. Berenson, R. J., Bensinger, W. I., Kalamasz, D., and Martin, P. (1986). Elimination of Daudi lymphoblasts from human bone marrow using avidin-biotin immunoadsorption. *Blood 67*:509.
31. Filipovich, A. H., Vallera, D. A., Youle, R. J., Quinones, R. R., Neville, D. M., and Kersey, J. H. (1984). Ex-vivo treatment of donor bone marrow with anti-T cell immunotoxins for prevention of graft-versus-host disease. *Lancet i*:469.
32. Casellas, P., Canat, X., Fauser, A. A., Gros, O., Laurent, G., Poncelet, P., and Jansen, F. K. (1985). Optimal elimination of leukemic T cells from human bone marrow with T101-ricin A chain immunotoxin. *Blood 65*:289.

33. Stong, R. C., Youle, R. J., and Vallera, D. A. (1984). Elimination of clono-
    genic T-leukemic cells from human bone marrow using anti-Mr 65,000 pro-
    tein immunotoxins. *Cancer Res. 44*:3000.
34. Myers, C. D., Thorpe, P. E., Ross, W. C. J., Cumber, A. J., Katz, F. E., Tax,
    W., and Greaves, M. F. (1984). An immunotoxin with therapeutic potential
    in T cell leukemia: WT1-Ricin A. *Blood 63*:1178.
35. Muirhead, M., Martin, P. J., Torok-Storb, B., Uhr, J. W., and Vitetta, E. S.
    (1983). Use of an antibody-ricin A-chain conjugate to delete neoplastic B
    cells from human bone marrow. *Blood 62*:327.
36. Coombes, R. C., Buckman, R., Forster, J. A., Shepherd, V., O'Hare, M. J.,
    Vincent, M., Powles, T. J., and Neville, A. M. (1986). In vitro and in vivo
    effects of a monoclonal antibody-toxin conjugate for use in autologous
    bone marrow transplantation for patients with breast cancer. *Cancer Res.
    46*:4217.
37. Uckun, F. M., Ramakrishnan, S., and Houston, L. L. (1985). Increased ef-
    ficiency in selective elimination of leukemia cells by a combination of stable
    derivative of cyclophosphamide and a human B-cell-specific immunotoxin
    containing pokeweed antiviral protein. *Cancer Res. 45*:69.
38. Ramakrishnan, S., and Houston, L. L. (1984). Inhibition of human acute
    lymphoblastic leukemia cells by immunotoxins: potentiation by chloro-
    quine. *Science 223*:58.
39. Bjorn, M. J., Groetsema, G., and Scalapino, L. (1986). Antibody-Pseudo-
    monas exotoxin A conjugates cytotoxic to human breast cancer cells in
    vitro. *Cancer Res. 46*:3262.
40. Martin, P. J., Hansen, J. A., and Viletta, E. S. (1985). A ricin A chain-con-
    taining immunotoxin that kills human T lymphocytes in vitro. *Blood 66*:
    908.
41. Economou, J. S., Shin, H. S., Kaizer, H., Santos, G. W., and Schron, D. S.
    (1978). Bone marrow transplantation in cancer therapy: inactivation by
    antibody and complement of tumor cells in mouse syngeneic marrow trans-
    plants (40223). *Proc. Soc. Exp. Biol. Med. 158*:449.
42. Feeney, M., Knapp, R. C., Greenberger, J. S., and Bast, J. C., Jr. (1981).
    Elimination of leukemic cells from rat bone marrow using antibody and
    complement. *Cancer Res. 41*:3331.
43. Hagenbeek, A., and Van Bekkum, D. W. (eds.) (1977). Proceedings of an
    International Workshop on "Comparative evaluation of the L5222 and the
    BNML rat leukemia models and their relevance for human acute leukemia."
    Leukemia Res. 1:75.
44. Gee, A. P., Rolfe, A. E., Wothington-White, D., Graham-Pole, J., and Boyle,
    M. D. (1985). A rapid alternative to the clonogenic assay for measuring
    antibody and complement-mediated killing of tumor cells. *Clin. Immunol.
    Immunopathol. 34*:263.
45. Uckun, R. M., Ramakrishnan, S., Haag, D., and Houston, L. L. (1985). Ex
    vivo elimination of lymphoblastic leukemia cells from human marrow by
    mafosfamid. *Leukemia Res. 9*:83.

46. Reynolds, C. P., Black, A. T., and Woody, J. N. (1986). Sensitive method for detecting viable cells seeded into bone marrow. *Cancer Res. 46*:5878.
47. Philip, I., Favrot, M. C., and Philip, T. (1987). Use of a liquid cell culture assay to quantify the elimination of Burkitt lymphoma cells from the bone marrow. *J. Immunol. Meth. 97*:11.
48. Ajani, J. A., Spitzer, G., Tomasovic, B., Drewinko, B., Hug, V. M., and Dicke, K. (1986). In vitro cytotoxicity patterns of standard and investigational agents on human bone marrow granulocyte-macrophage progenitor cells. *Br. J. Cancer 54*:607.
49. Uckun, F. M., Gajil-Peczalska, K. J., Kersey, J. H., Houston, L. L., and Vallera, D. A. (1986). Use of a novel colony assay to evaluate the cytotoxicity of an immunotoxin containing pokeweed antiviral protein against blast progenitor cells freshly obtained from patients with common B-lineage acute lymphoblastic leukemia. *J. Exp. Med. 163*:347.
50. Campana, D., and Janossy, G. (1986). Leukemia diagnosis and testing of complement fixing antibodies for bone marrow purging in acute lymphoid leukemia. *Blood 68*:1264.
51. Moss, T. J., Seeger, R. C., Kindler-Rohrborn, A., Marangos, P. J., Rajevsky, M. F., and Reynolds, C. P. (1985). Immunohistologic detection and phenotyping of neuroblastoma cells in bone marrow using cytoplasmic neuron specific enolase and cell surface antigens. *Adv. Neuroblast. Res. 175*:367.
52. Laurent, G., Kuhlein, E., Casellas, P., Canat, X., Carayon, P., Poncelet, P., Correll, S., Rigal, F., and Jansen, F. K. (1986). Determination of sensitivity of fresh leukemia cells to immunotoxins. *Cancer Res. 46*:2289.
53. Philip, I., Philip, T., Favrot, M. C., Vuillaume, M., Fontanière, B., Chamard, D., and Lenoir, G. M. (1984). Establishment of lymphomatous cell lines from bone marrow samples from patients with Burkitt's lymphoma. *J. Natl. Cancer Inst. 73*:835.
54. Philip, L., Favrot, M. C., Combaret, V., Laurent, J. C., Kremens, B., and Philip, T. (1986). Use of a liquid cell culture assay to measure the in vitro Burkitt cell elimination from the BM in preclinical and clinical procedures. *Proceedings of the Second International Symposium on ABMT*, Houston. In press.
55. Philip, T., Bernard, J. L., Zucker, J. M., Pinkerton, R., Lutz, P., Bordigoni, P., Plouvier, E., Robert, A., Carton, R., Philippe, N., Philip, I., and Favrot, M. C. (1987). High dose chemotherapy with bone marrow transplantation as consolidation treatment in neuroblastoma: an unselected group of stage IV patients over one year of age. *J. Clin. Oncol. 5*:266.
56. Kemshead, J. T., Heath, L., Gibson, F. M., Katz, F., Richmond, F., Trealaven, J., and Ugelstad, J. (1986). Magnetic microspheres and monoclonal antibodies for the depletion of neuroblastoma cells from bone marrow: experiences, improvements and observations. *Br. J. Cancer 54*:771.
57. De Fabriitis, P., Bregni, M., Lipton, J., Greenberger, J., Nadler, L., Rothstein, L., Korbling, M., Ritz, J., and Bast, R. C. (1985). Elimination of clonogenic Burkitt's lymphoma cells from human bone marrow using 4-

hydroxyperoxycyclophosphamide in combination with monoclonal antibodies and complement. *Blood 5*:1064.

58. Lebien, T. W., Anderson, J. M., Vallera, D. A., and Uckun, F. M. (1986). Increased efficacy in selective elimination of leukemic cell line clonogenic cells by a combination of monoclonal antibodies BA-1, BA-2, BA-3 + complement and mafosfamid (ASTA Z 7557). *Leukemia Res. 10*:139.

59. Favrot, M. C., Philip, I., Poncelet, P., Combaret, V., Kremens, B., Janossy, G., and Philip, T. (1986). Comparative efficiency of an immunomagnetic procedure and a rabbit complement lysis to eliminate BL cells from the bone marrow. *Proceedings of the Second International Symposium on ABMT*, Houston. In press.

60. Chang, J., Coutinho, L., Morgenstein, G., Scarffe, J. H., Deakin, D., Harrison, C., Testa, N. G., and Dexter, T. M. (1986). Reconstitution of haemopoietic system with autologous marrow taken during relapse of acute myeloblastic leukaemia and grown in long-term culture. *Lancet 8*:294.

61. Berenson, R. J., Andrews, R. G., Bensinger, W. I., Kalamasz, D., Knitter, G., and Bernstein, I. D. (1986). In vivo reconstitution of hematopoiesis in baboons using 12.8 positive marrow cells isolated by avidin-biotin immunoadsorption (abstr. 1025). *Blood 68*:287.

62. Reiffers, J., Bernard, P., David, B., Vezon, G., Sarrat, A., Marit, G., Moulinier, J., and Broustet, A. (1986). Successful autologous transplantation with peripheral blood hepopoietic cells in a patient with acute leukemia. *Exp. Hematol. 14*:312.

63. To, L. B., Haylock, D. N., Kimber, R. J., and Juttner, C. A. (1984). High levels of circulating haematopoiesis stem cells in very early remission from acute non-lymphoblastic leukaemia and their collection and cryopreservation. *Br. J. Haematol. 58*:399.

64. Rosenberg, S. A., Lotze, M. T., Muul, L. M., Leitman, S., Chang, A. E., Ettinghausen, S. E., Matory, Y. L., Skibber, J. M., Shiloni, E., Vetto, J. T., Seipp, G. A., Simpson, C., and Reichert, C. M. (1985). Observations on the systemic administration of autologous lymphokine-activated killer cells and recombinant interleukin-2 to patients with metastatic cancer. *N. Engl. J. Med. 313*:1485.

65. Bast, R. C., Jr., Sallan, S. E., Reynolds, C., Lipton, J., and Ritz, J. (1985). Autologous bone marrow transplantation for CALLA-positive acute lymphoblastic leukemia: an update. In *Autologous Bone Marrow Transplantation*. Edited by K. A. Dicke, G. Spitzer, and A. R. Zander. Houston, pp. 3–6.

66. Ramsay, N., Lebien, T. W., Nesbit, M., McGlave, P., Weisdorf, D., Kenyon, P., Hurd, D., Goldman, A., Kim, T., and Kersey, J. (1985). Autologous bone marrow transplantation for patients with acute lymphoblastic leukemia in second or subsequent remission. Results of bone marrow related with monoclonal antibodies BA-1, BA-2 and BA-3 plus complement. *Blood 66*:508.

67. Nadler, L. M., Takvorian, T., Botnick, L., Bast, R. C., Finberg, R., Hellman, S., Canellos, G. P., and Schlossman, S. F. (1984). Anti-B$_1$ monoclonal antibody and complement treatment in autologous bone marrow transplantation for relapsed B-cell non-Hodgkin's lymphoma. *Lancet 25*:427.
68. Forster, H. K., Obrecht, J. P., Knaak, T., Baumgartner, C., Wagner, H. P., and Gudat, F. G. (1984). Use of a monoclonal anti-human B-cell antibody in diagnosis and therapy of non-Hodgkin's lymphoma. In *Leucocyte Typing*. Edited by A. Bernard, L. Baumsell, L. Dausset, C. Milstein, and S. Schlossman. Springer Verlag, Berlin, pp. 614–618.
69. Baumgartner, C., Brun del Re, G., Forster, H. K., Bucher, U., Delaveu, B., Hirt, A., Imbach, P., Luthy, A., Stern, A. C., and Wagner, H. P. (1985). Autologous bone marrow transplantation for pediatric non-Hodgkin's lymphoma: in vitro purging of the graft with anti-Y29/55 monoclonal antibody and complement. In *Autologous Bone Marrow Transplantation*. Edited by K. A. Dicke, G. Spitzer, and A. R. Zander. Houston, pp. 377–381.
70. Philip, T., Bernard, J. L., Zucker, J. M., Pinkerton, R., Lutz, P., Bordigoni, P., Plouvier, E., Robert, A., Carton, R., Philippe, N., Philip, I., and Favrot, M. C. (1987). High dose chemotherapy with bone marrow transplantation as consolidation treatment in neuroblastoma: an unselected group of stage IV patients over one year of age. *J. Clin. Oncol. 5*:266–271.
71. Seeger, R. C., Wells, J., Lenarsky, C., Feig, S. A., Selch, M., Moss, T. J., Ugelstad, J., and Reynolds, C. P. (1986). Bone marrow transplantation for poor prognosis neuroblastoma (abstr. 20). *J. Cell Biochem. 10D*:215.
72. Douay, L., Gorin, N. C., Laporte, J. P., Lopez, M., Najman, A., and Duhamel, G. (1984). ASTA Z 7557 (INN mafosfamide) for the in vitro treatment of human leukemic bone marrows. *Invest. New Drugs 2*:187.

8

Diagnostic and Therapeutic Procedures with Haptens and Glycoproteins (Antigens and Antibodies) Coupled Covalently by Specific Sites to Insoluble Supports

GERARD A. QUASH, VINCENT THOMAS, GEORGES OGIER,
SAID EL ALAOUI, JEAN-GUY DELCROS, HUGUETTE RIPOLL,
ANNE-MARIE ROCH, and STEPHANE LEGASTELOIS
Unité de Virologie—INSERM, Lyon, France

RICHARD GIBERT
Université Claude Bernard, Lyon, France

JEAN-PIERRE RIPOLL
Hôpital Cardiovasculaire et Pneumologique, Lyon, France

I. INTRODUCTION

Antigens and antibodies *adsorbed* to insoluble supports such as red blood cells, polystyrene (latex) particles, nylon spheres, polystyrene or polyvinyl microtiter plates, nitrocellulose, and nylon membranes are routinely used in diagnostic procedures such as agglutination tests, enzyme-linked immunosorbent assays (ELISA), and radioimmunoassays (RIA).

Examples of antigens and antibodies *covalently* coupled to insoluble supports such as functionalized polysaccharide and nylon matrices for the chromatographic purification of the corresponding immunoreactive partner are also well documented. However, covalently bound antigens and antibodies have not met with widespread acceptance in diagnostic procedures.

All the various reasons which can be put forward to explain the delay in adopting covalent coupling for diagnostic purposes can be summed up in one statement: "Do covalently coupled products offer any intrinsic advantage over adsorbed products?"

155

Table 1 Stokes Radius of BSA and of IgG Adsorbed to Polystyrene Latex Spheres

	Approximate ellipsoid dimensions Å		Stokes' radius Å	Differences in Stokes' radii
	BSA	IgG		
Latex	—	—	823 ± 16	—
BSA	140X38X38	—	861 ± 2	38
IgG	—	235X44X44	1033 ± 20	210

Source: Data taken from Refs. 1 and 2.

To perceive the improvements which could be brought about by covalent coupling we must first summarize the problems encountered on immobilizing proteins.

A. Protein Immobilization

1. Problems with Adsorption

Thanks to the work of many authors (1,2) it is well established that the adsorption of bovine serum albumin (BSA) and of human immunoglobulin (IgG) to polystyrene surfaces takes place *side-on* for BSA and *end-on* for IgG (Table 1). Further, Morrissey and Han (2) have suggested that at low ligand to support ratio BSA undergoes flattening which could induce distortion of some of its antigenic sites. For proteins which are adsorbed side-on (BSA) there could occur a loss of reactivity at those epitopes which are directly in contact with the insoluble support and also at those which have been distorted by the adsorption procedure. The importance of these phenomena could not be fully appreciated when polyclonal antibodies were used because there would always have remained epitopes which had retained sufficient activity to interact with their corresponding antibodies present in the heterogenous polyclonal antibody population. At present, with the increasing widespread use of adsorbed antigens for screening monoclonal antibodies (MAb), there is the distinct possibility that hidden or distorted epitopes may not interact with a particular MAb.

2. Theoretical Advantages of Site-Specific Covalent Coupling

One criterion which can be immediately laid down for covalent coupling is that it should *preserve the configuration* of epitopes on the immobilized antigen. However, when the functional group by which the antigen is to be attached is itself involved in the integrity of the antigenic site, then the antigen must be immobilized by other functional groups. Another criterion which covalent coupling must therefore satisfy is that of *site-specific attachment*.

B. Enunciation of Topics to be Presented

This presentation will not include generally available methods for covalently coupling proteins which have been extensively reviewed. We will instead:

a. Summarize methods for the site-specific covalent coupling of glyco-proteins via their carbohydrate or protein residues (see Sect. II.A and B)

b. Provide evidence that the antibody titer obtained with site-specifically coupled viral antigens gives a better indication of the clinical status (e.g., neutralizing antibody titer) of a patient than that obtained with ad-sorbed antigen (see Sect. III.A to D)

c. Show that covalently bound reagents permit the development of proced-ures for removing high-molecular weight constituents from plasma (see Sect. II.A.6) and for measuring the titer of specific antibodies in immuno-complexes (see Sect. IV.A to D)

II. EXPERIMENTAL PROCEDURES FOR SITE-SPECIFIC COVALENT COUPLING

In all cases, only the principles will be outlined, experimental details can be found in the corresponding references.

A. Functionalized Latex Spheres as the Insoluble Support

1. Insertion of Side Arms on to Carboxylated Latex (Rhone-Poulenc, France; Polysciences, West Germany)

To carboxylated latex spheres with diameters from 0.3 μm to 1.5 μm, an ali-phatic side arm, hexamethylenediamine (HMD) was first linked by a peptide bond using a water-soluble carbodiimide (3,4). The terminal amine group was then substituted with glutaraldehyde at an alkaline pH (5). Excess glutaralde-hyde was removed by washing, after which the terminal aldehyde group was substituted with adipic dihydrazide (ADH).

After elimination of the excess dihydrazide, the latex spheres with substi-tuted side arms were reduced with a reducing agent (e.g., $NaBH_3CN$) in order to stabilize the Schiff's base formed between the primary amine group of HMD and the aldehyde group of glutaraldehyde. A schematic representation of this substitution is shown in Figure 1.

However, glutaraldehyde at an alkaline pH undergoes aldol condensation to form polymers (6) (Fig. 2) so that depending on the degree of polymerization,

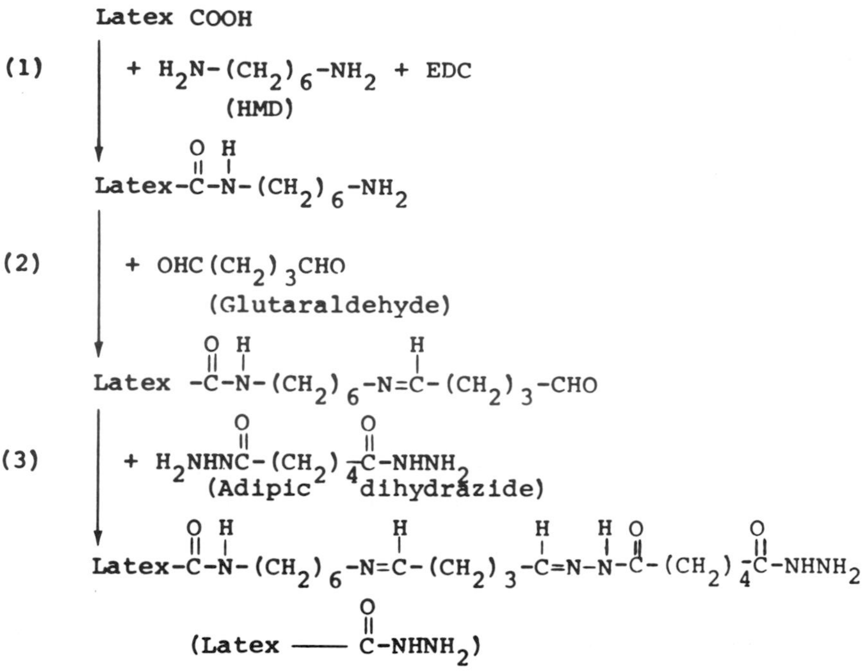

```
     Latex COOH
(1)  |   + H₂N-(CH₂)₆-NH₂ + EDC
     |       (HMD)
     ↓         O H
               ‖ |
         Latex-C-N-(CH₂)₆-NH₂

(2)  |   + OHC(CH₂)₃CHO
     |       (Glutaraldehyde)
     ↓         O H              H
               ‖ |              |
         Latex -C-N-(CH₂)₆-N=C-(CH₂)₃-CHO

(3)  |         O              O
     |         ‖              ‖
     |   + H₂NHNC-(CH₂)₄C-NHNH₂
     |       (Adipic dihydrazide)
     ↓
         O H              H       H H O              O
         ‖ |              |       | | ‖              ‖
   Latex-C-N-(CH₂)₆-N=C-(CH₂)₃-C=N-N-C-(CH₂)₄C-NHNH₂

                         O
                         ‖
         (Latex ——— C-NHNH₂)
```

Figure 1 Preparation of latex spheres with acid hydrazide end groups according to the reaction sequence: hexamethylene diamine (HMD), glutaraldehyde, and adipic dihydrazide.

the insoluble support is in fact substituted by a polyglutaraldehyde side arm containing many branched chain free aldehyde groups.

These free carbonyls provide sites for the attachment of ADH previously used, or for the attachment of markers or ligands with free amine groups. Ligand binding is therefore indiscriminate and may involve multiple binding sites per molecule with the ensuing risk of distortion.

To overcome this problem of glutaraldehyde polymerization, substitution after HMD insertion was continued using succinic anhydride followed by derivatization of the terminal carboxyl group to an acid hydrazide using hydrazine hydrate and a water-soluble carbodiimide (7). Figure 3 summarizes this procedure.

2. Insertion of Side Arms on to Aminated Latex
   (Advanced Magnetics, USA; Sintef, Norway)

In the case of aminated latex spheres, the primary amine groups were directly derivatized with succinic anhydride and then the terminal carboxyl group was

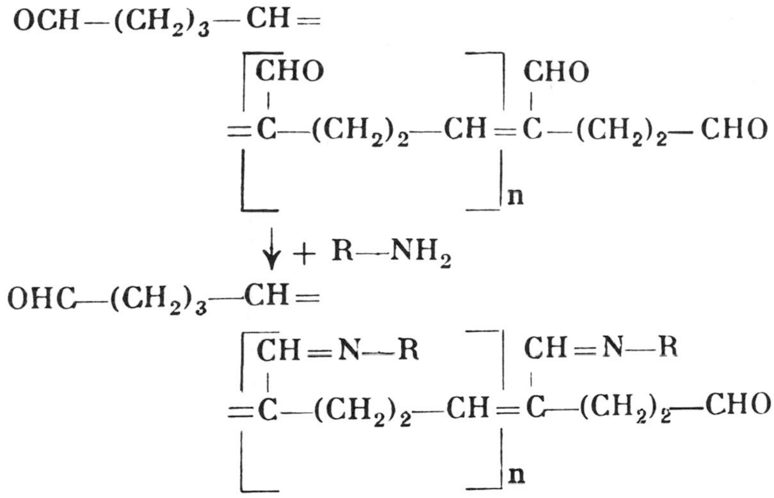

$$OCH-(CH_2)_3-CH=$$

$$\left[\begin{array}{c} CHO \\ | \\ =C-(CH_2)_2-CH= \end{array}\right] \begin{array}{c} CHO \\ | \\ C-(CH_2)_2-CHO \end{array}$$

$$\downarrow + R-NH_2$$

$$OHC-(CH_2)_3-CH=$$

$$\left[\begin{array}{c} CH=N-R \\ | \\ =C-(CH_2)_2-CH= \end{array}\right] \begin{array}{c} CH=N-R \\ | \\ C-(CH_2)_2-CHO \end{array}$$

Figure 2 Diagram taken from Monzan et al. (6).

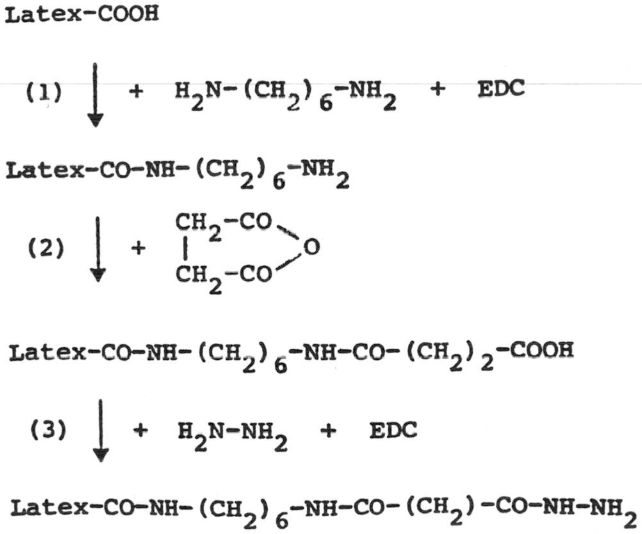

Latex-COOH

(1) $\downarrow$ + $H_2N-(CH_2)_6-NH_2$ + EDC

Latex-CO-NH-$(CH_2)_6$-NH$_2$

(2) $\downarrow$ + $\begin{array}{c} CH_2-CO \\ | \\ CH_2-CO \end{array}\!\!\!\diagup O$

Latex-CO-NH-$(CH_2)_6$-NH-CO-$(CH_2)_2$-COOH

(3) $\downarrow$ + H_2N-NH_2 + EDC

Latex-CO-NH-$(CH_2)_6$-NH-CO-(CH_2)-CO-NH-NH$_2$

Figure 3 Preparation of latex spheres with acid hydrazide end groups according to the reaction sequence: hexamethylene diamine, succinic anhydride, and hydrazine.

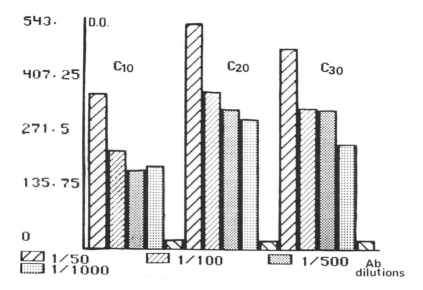

Figure 4 Goat IgG anti-mouse IgG (GAM) was coupled via its carbohydrate residues to terminal acid hydrazides on magnetic spheres substituted with C10, C20, and C30 side arms. The *accessibility* of antigenic sites on GAM was measured by its reaction with different dilutions of a rabbit serum anti-goat IgG (RAG) labeled with alkaline phosphatase. Determination of alkaline phosphatase activity showed that at all dilutions used, GAM on a C20 side arm reacts better than GAM on C10 or on C30 side arms.

converted to acid hydrazide as described in the preceding section. The number of acid hydrazide groups was determined by diazotation and by hydrazone formation. With Sintef magnetic spheres, 2.23 nmol [^{14}C] ethanolamine were bound by amide bonds, and 12.58 nmol [^{14}C] pyruvate by hydrazone bonds per milligram spheres.

3. Determination of the Optimum Length of the Side Arm

The work of Cuatrecasas and Anfinsen (8) has established that the efficient interaction of an enzyme with its immobilized substrate depends on the length of the side arm separating the substrate from the insoluble support. We therefore undertook the determination of the optimum length of the aliphatic side arm necessary for the retention of the native configuration and reactivity of goat IgG anti-mouse IgG (GAM). The GAM was coupled to terminal acid hydrazides via its carbohydrate residues which had been oxidized as previously described (9). Native configuration was assessed by measuring the accessibility of antigenic sites of the coupled GAM to a rabbit serum anti-goat IgG labeled with

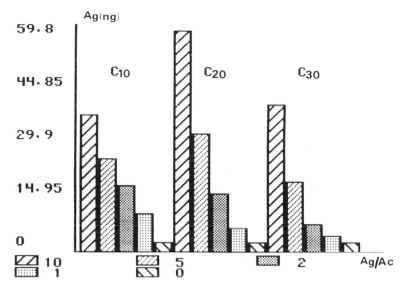

Figure 5 Goat IgG anti-mouse IgG (GAM) was coupled via its carbohydrate residues to terminal acid hydrazides on magnetic spheres substituted with C10, C20, and C30 side arms. The *reactivity* of bound GAM was assessed with [^{3}II]-labeled mouse IgG at four different ratios of mouse IgG/GAM. Determination of the radioactivity bound to the spheres showed that GAM on C20 side arms was the most reactive.

alkaline phosphatase. Reactivity was measured by the interaction of the coupled Ab with [^{3}H]-labeled mouse IgG. The specificity of interaction was controlled using another aliquot of acid hydrazide-derivatized spheres but coupled instead to goat IgG anti-human IgG.

Figure 4 shows that the antigenic sites on goat IgG at the end of a C20 side arm are more accessible to rabbit anti-goat IgG than those on a C10 or a C30 side arm. Figure 5 shows that the reactivity of the Fab portion on the C20 side arm was also greater than that on the C10 or the C30.

Taken together these results confirm those reported by O'Shanessy and Quarles (10) that the insertion of a side arm between the insoluble support and the carbohydrate portion of the Ab increases the immunoreactivity of carbohydrate-bound antibody.

4. Site-Specific Coupling of Glycoproteins

Terminal acid hydrazides are versatile functionalities in that:

1. They can react with the carbonyl groups of oxidized carbohydrates of glycoproteins to form stable hydrazones

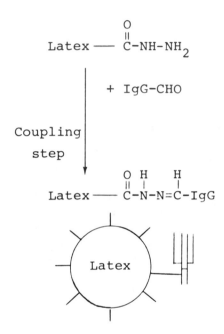

IgG + NaIO$_4$ ⟶ IgG-CHO

Figure 6 Schematic representation of the oxidation of IgG and its coupling via the aldehydes generated to acid hydrazide groups at the end of a side-arm attached to latex spheres.

2. They can be diazotized with nitrous acid to give acid azides which form peptide bonds with free amino groups (N terminal or ε amino groups of lysine) on proteins.

(a) Hydrazone Formation with Glycoproteins: In the examples given previously the antibodies were coupled by hydrazones formed between the terminal acid hydrazide on the support and aldehyde groups generated by the action of periodate on carbohydrates which are situated primarily on the CH$_2$ region of the Fc portion of the Ab molecule. This is represented schematically in Figure 6. However, IgG molecules with carbohydrates on light chains have been reported (11). Even in these instances, hydrazone formation would be beneficial since the amino acid residues in the Fab portion would be left intact.

Table 2 Ratio of Surface Areas of H & L Chains of Human IgG After Separation by PAGE

	Surface area		Ratio of surface area:
	H	L	H/L
Free IgG	679.5	869.5	0.78
IgG linked by peptide bonds (carbodiimide)	515	722	0.71
IgG linked by hydrazone bonds	199	569.5	0.35

Free human IgG and latex with bound human IgG were treated directly with β mercaptoethanol and SDS for 5 min at 95°C and then separated by electrophoresis on 9% polyacrylamide gels. Gels were stained with silver nitrate and the surface areas of the stained bands were integrated on a Vernon photometer integrating densitometer.

(b) Evidence for the Preferential Coupling of Human IgG Via H Chains: Is there any evidence for the site-specific coupling of IgG via H chains or is IgG coupled indiscriminately via hydrazone formation with carbohydrates on H and L chains? The results presented in Table 2 show that the treatment of the IgG-bound latex with β-mercaptoethanol for 5 min at 95°C followed by the separation of the reduced products on polyacrylamide gel electrophoresis (PAGE) and silver nitrate staining yields a ratio of H to L chains of approximately 0.35. On the contrary, with free IgG or with IgG coupled to latex spheres by peptide bonds, similar treatment yields a ratio of H to L of about 0.78.

This diminution in the proportion of H to L chains after hydrazone formation provides evidence for the preferential coupling of IgG molecules via their H chains.

(c) Peptide Bond Formation with Glycoproteins: Peptide bond formation between diazotized acid hydrazide groups on latex spheres and ϵ amino groups of fetuin was undertaken to preserve the integrity of carbohydrate residues on this protein and in particular terminal sialic acid residues. Because of its high content of sialic acid, fetuin is routinely used as a substrate for neuraminidases of cellular and viral origin such as influenza virus.

The method presently recommended by WHO (12) for characterizing the neuraminidases of influenza viruses and for titrating neuraminidase antibodies

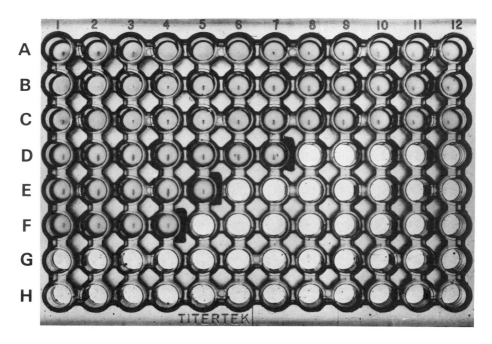

Figure 7 (A) MRC11 serial dilutions from 1/20 onward; (B) A/Bangkok/1/79 serial dilutions from 1/10 onward; (C) Heq$_1$ N Vic 75 serial dilutions from 1/10 onward; (D) Control allantoic fluid; E, Fetuin latex control; H, unused wells.

consists of incubating influenza virus preparations with fetuin for 18 h at 37°C, and then determining the amount of released sialic acid by oxidation with periodate followed by the thiobarbituric acid procedure of Warren (13). The entire procedure takes approximately 24 h, employs many different reagents, and is long, laborious, and expensive. It is thus ill-adapted to routine analysis. We therefore tried to develop reagents and simple technical procedures which would permit the detection of neuraminidase.

For simplicity of operation, an agglutination test in which latex spheres were the solid support seemed appropriate. Such an agglutination test would have the advantage of detecting directly the enzyme substrate complex without the need to measure the product of the reaction sialic acid.

5. Quantitative Test Procedures with Covalently Bound Ligands

(a) Visual Agglutination Tests with Glycoproteins: Latex spheres with bound fetuin (38 μg/mg latex) were prepared as described and a Fetuin Latex Agglutination Test (FLAT) procedure was developed (14).

Figure 7 shows the results obtained when fetuin latex spheres were mixed with the allantoic fluid from infected embryonated eggs. In some instances a zone phenomenon was observed as in row A with a recombinant virus MRC 11−$H_3 N_2$ 73; row C with Heq_1 NVic 75−Heq_1 N_2 75 but not in row B with A/Bangkok/1/79−$H_3 N_2$ 79. Rows D, E, and F contained, respectively, control noninfected allantoic fluid, the glycine NaOH BSA pluriol buffer used for the reaction and latex fetuin in NaCl glycine-NaOH buffer.

It is noteworthy that regardless of whether the hemagglutinin is from a proto-type or recombinant strain, the fetuin latex spheres were agglutinated. This ob-servation provides strong evidence for the interaction of latex-bound fetuin with viral neuraminidase specifically.

With the same latex-fetuin spheres, the titer of anti-influenza virus neuramini-dase antibodies in sera was determined by FLAT inhibition in microtiter plates (15).

Latex-rabbit IgG antifibrin degradation products (FDP) have been used for measuring FDP in sera by a slide agglutination procedure (9).

Latex-measles virus coupled via its carbohydrate moieties was used for titer-ing antimeasles antibodies in sera by agglutination in microtiter plates (9).

(b) Nephelometric Assays with a Hapten:Putrescine: In addition to the above-mentioned test systems latex spheres with a bound hapten-putrescine have been used in nephelometry (16). Figure 8 shows that, depending on the number of molecules of polyamine bound per sphere, the reaction is different. For example in the presence of spheres with 20 nmol of putrescine/mg latex, no signal is obtained on nephelometry. With spheres containing 1.7 pmol/mg the signal is still very weak, and with spheres containing 600 pmol/mg the signal is well defined. The response on nephelometry is strictly dependent on the stoich-iometry of coupling.

6. Qualitative Experimental Approach with Covalently
    Bound Glycoproteins

(a) Scanning Electron Microscopy: Latex spheres with fetuin bound via its *protein* residues have been used for detecting neuraminidase sites on the surface of cells infected with fowl plague virus (17). Latex spheres with rabbit IgG anti-polyamine bound via their *carbohydrate* moieties permitted polyamine sites on the surface of transformed cells to be visualized (18).

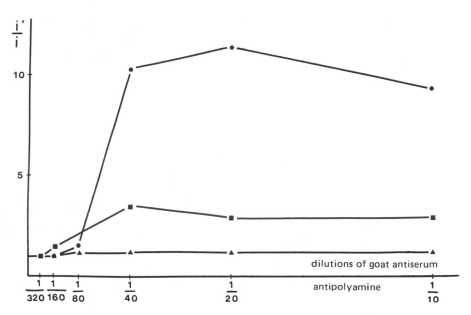

Figure 8 Light scattered by latex-PUT spheres (1) alone and (1') in the presence of antiserum: (■): 1.7, (●), 600, (▲): 20,000 pmol PUT/mg latex.

(b) Apheresis for the Selective Removal of Protein-Bound Polyamines from the Plasma of Tumor-Bearing Mice: One further application of covalently bound antibodies but this time to magnetic latex, is in apheresis. A variation of this procedure is currently used in clinical situations such as bone marrow purging (19,20). In view of our previous observations showing that the plasma from cancer patients contains bound polyamines (21), we employed magnetic latex spheres with carbohydrate coupled antipolyamine antibodies to try to isolate these protein-bound polyamines from the plasma of mice grafted with the Lewis lung carcinoma.

It is apparent from the densitometer tracings of Figure 9 that protein-bound polyamines can indeed be isolated from the plasma of mice. Three proteins of MW 27, 55, and 82K were isolated from the plasma of normal mice. In mice bearing the Lewis lung carcinoma from the first week after tumor graft, polyamines were carried by at least eight other proteins of higher MW. These eight proteins were not isolated if the magnetic spheres with bound antipolyamine antibodies were preincubated with carrier-bound spermine, nor were they present in the plasma of mice in which inflammation and hypertrophy were induced by the injection of heat-inactivated *Brucella abortus* (22).

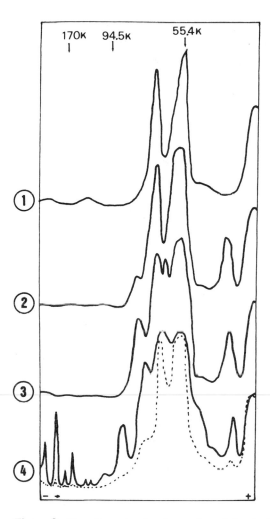

Figure 9   Densitometer tracings of proteins isolated by latex bound antipolyamine antibodies (immunolatex) after incubation with: buffer alone (1), or
plasmas: from normal mice (2), from mice infected with *Brucella abortus* (3),
from mice bearing the Lewis lung carcinoma 3 weeks after the graft (4).
4- - - - -: immunolatex preincubated with carrier-bound spermine before addition of plasma from mice 3 weeks after tumor graft. Separation on 9% polyacrylamide gel.

The extension of this approach to other constituents in plasma can be readily envisaged using, for example, monoclonal antibodies.

The foregoing examples show quite clearly the experimental approach used and the results obtained when glycoproteins covalently bound to latex spheres interact directly with their corresponding biologically reactive partner. However with agglutination, the limit of detection is dependent on the stoichiometry of coupling (see Sect. II.A.5), the avidity of the antibody and the rapidity with which results must be obtained.

To increase sensitivity, we therefore decided to develop enzyme immunoassays using covalently bound antigens and antibodies.

B. Functionalized Polystyrene Microtiter Plates, Nylon, and Cellulose Acetate Strips ad the Insoluble Support

1. Preparation of Polyhydrazidostyrene Microtiter Plates

Polystyrene plates were first nitrated with a v/v mixture 47/53 concentrated nitric and sulfuric acids for 5 min at 4°C as described by Chin and Links (23). At the end of this period the polynitrostyrene plates were washed extensively with deionized water and then reduced for 6 h at 60°C under vacuum with a mixture of 6% sodium dithionite in solution in $2M$ KOH. The number of amino groups inserted on to the polystyrene was determined by their reactivity with picryl sulfonic acid in the presence of saturated borate pH 10. O.D. measurements (using a MR 580 Microelisa Auto Reader Dynatech) were carried out at 405 nm on wells randomly distributed over one plate from each batch. These gave values for amino group substitution of 0.258 ± 0.037 (n=12). For six different batches, this value was 0.225 ± 0.033. Polyaminostyrene plates were then suspended in 50 mM borate buffer pH 9 and treated with solid succinic anhydride. After two consecutive treatments the plates were washed with deionized water and the terminal carboxyl groups were converted to acid hydrazide using a water-soluble carbodiimide and hydrazine hydrate. The extent of hydrazine substitution was assessed with picryl sulfonic acid and the number of acid hydrazide groups was determined by amide formation with [^{14}C]ethanolamine. There were on an average around 110 nmol acid hydrazide functionalities per well.

2. Chemical Substitution of Aminated Nylon Strips

When aminated nylon was used as the insoluble support, it was first directly succinylated and then converted to acid hydrazide as described for aminostyrene.

3. Chemical Substitution of Nitrocellulose Strips

In the case of nitrocellulose, the support was first oxidized by sodium periodate then treated directly with adipic dihydrazide and further reduced with

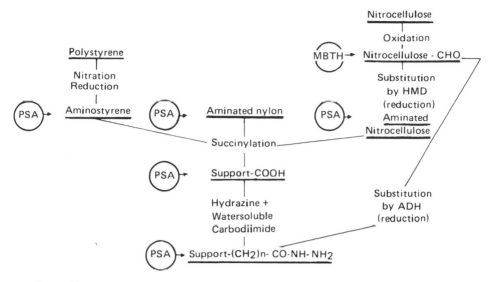

Figure 10 ADH: adipic dihydrazide; MBTH: 3-methyl-2-benzothiazolinone hydrazone; PSA: picryl sulfonic acid.

sodium borohydride. Figure 10 summarizes the different substitution steps and verification procedures with these three supports. For further details see Quash (24).

Nylon acid hydrazide and nitrocellulose acid hydrazide were diazotized and used for covalently binding proteins such as protein A and casein by peptide bonds. Further, spermine could be linked via peptide bonds to free carboxyl groups on the casein already bound. Diazotized nitrocellulose strips were also used for covalently binding DNA (24).

Onto these nylon acid hydrazide strips, immunoglobulins with oxidized carbohydrates could also be coupled via hydrazone formation. Using labeled immunoglobulin, it was possible to calculate that the maximum binding capacity of a nylon strip was about 1.5 μg/mm^2.

4. Quantitative Test Procedure (ELISA) on PHS Plates

Once the chemistry for covalent coupling on these strips and microtiter plates had been worked out and the coupled molecules were shown to have retained their biological activity, we were able to undertake enzyme immunoassays which allowed us to formulate the general question asked in the Introduction in precise terms.

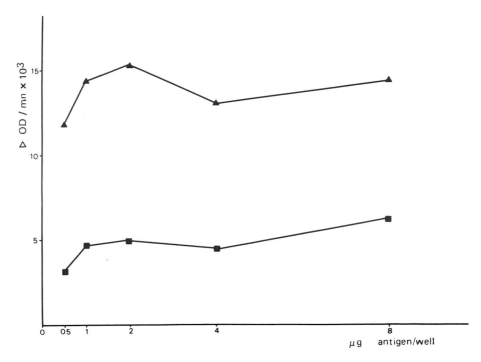

Figure 11 Human IgG was measured by its reaction with a goat serum anti-human Fc labeled with alkaline phosphatase. (▲) amine-coupled CMV (NH$_2$ ELISA); (■) carbohydrate-coupled CMV (OCA ELISA).

(a) Do Glycoprotein Antigens Which Are Covalently Bound to Insoluble Supports by Their Amino Acid or Their Carbohydrate Residues React Differently with a Serum Containing a Heterogenous Population of Antibodies?:
This question was all the more important for viral glycoproteins since viruses contain genetic information for their proteins but not for their carbohydrate residues. The type and sequence of carbohydrate residues are determined by the host cell. Further, it has been shown that pretreatment of adenovirus 5 with periodate destroyed the hemagglutinin activity of the virus but not its capacity to elicit neutralizing antibody (25).

(b) Reply Using Cytomegalovirus (CMV) Glycoproteins on ELISA: To answer the question formulated above, chemically substituted microtiter plates with side arms terminating in either a carboxyl or acid hydrazide functionality were used to couple CMV virus, respectively, by the amino groups of lysine residues or by their carbohydrate residues which had been previously oxidized with periodate.

It is apparent (Fig. 11) that the reactivity of sera with anti-CMV antibodies is greater with CMV attached via its amino groups (NH_2 ELISA) than with CMV attached via its oxidized carbohydrate residues (OCA ELISA).

III. ANTIBODY TITERS BY BIOLOGICAL NEUTRALIZATION AND SEROLOGICAL DETERMINATION (ELISA)

A. Comparison Between Anti-CMV Titers Obtained by Adsorption ELISA, OCA ELISA, and Biological Neutralization

This was carried out on human IgG preparations containing anti-CMV antibody. The results obtained (Table 3) show that there is a better correlation between the titers obtained with carbohydrate-coupled antigens (OCA ELISA) and the neutralization titer than that obtained between the titers found with adsorbed antigens (adsorption ELISA) and the neutralization titer.

In view of these results, the question was asked whether the better correlation with neutralization obtained in the case of OCA ELISA was due to the coupling procedure per se or whether it was due to the carbohydrate oxidation step.

Table 3 Titers of CMV Antibodies in Purified Human IgG

Purified globulin no.	Titers determined by the ELISA adsorption method[a]	Titers determined by the neutralized method[b]	Titers determined by the covalent ELISA method
Y0504	67	128	50
Y0714	144	256	50
Y0880	519	256	100
Y0969	1087	512	400
Y1042	54	64	< 50
Y0741	67	128	50
Y0287	432	256	200
Y0417	2780	465	364
Y0454	1005	621	727
S1416	2923	512	400
Y0841	387	128	200
Y0896	593	256	100
Y1062	54	64	< 50
Y1094	455	256	50

[a]vs. br = 0.74
[b]vs. cr = 0.89

Table 4 Titers of CMV Antibodies in Purified Human IgG

IgG Sample	Neutralization titer	Ox Oligosaccharide Attached ELISA titer	Amine Attached Oligosaccharide Ox ELISA titer	Amine Attached ELISA titer	Adsorption ELISA titer
1	128	50	< 50	400	67
2	256	50	< 50	200	144
3	256	100	100	400	519
4	512	400	100	800	1087
5	64	< 50	< 50	50	54
6	128	50	50	200	67
7	256	200	200	800	432
8	465	364	181	727	2780
9	621	485	485	485	1005
10	512	400	400	> 1600	2923
11	128	200	100	400	387
12	256	100	100	1600	593
13	64	< 50	50	54	100
14	256	50	50	455	400

Table 5 Comparisons of Assays for CMV-Neutralizing Antibodies

Assay	Linear correlation coefficients				
	Neutralization	Adsorption ELISA attached	Ox Oligosaccharide ELISA	Amine-attached ELISA	Amine-attached oligosaccharide Ox ELISA
Neutralization	1				
Adsorption ELISA	0.74	1			
Ox Oligosaccharide-attached ELISA	0.90	0.75	1		
Amine-attached ELISA	0.52	0.62	0.41	1	
Amine-attached oligosaccharide Ox ELISA[a]	0.78 (0.87)	0.65 (0.64)	0.82 (0.93)	0.46 (0.48)	1

[a]The number in parentheses represents the correlation coefficient obtained when one aberrant titer value was discarded.

B. The Importance of Oxidized Carbohydrate Per Se Versus Oxidized and Coupled Carbohydrate to the OCA ELISA Titer

To answer this question, the following experimental approach was adopted. It consisted in immobilizing CMV virus by four different procedures:

1. Covalent coupling (amide bond formation with) amino acid residues but with no oxidation of the carbohydrate
2. Covalent coupling via the amino acid residues with subsequent oxidation of the carbohydrate
3. Coupling via hydrazone bonds with oxidized carbohydrate
4. Adsorbing the virus without any chemical modification

Viruses immobilized by each procedure were used to determine the antibody titers of IgG preparations containing anti CMV antibody. The results obtained are shown in Table 4.

When comparisons were made between the titers obtained by the different procedures and the neutralization antibody titer, it was apparent again that the best correlation with the neutralization antibody titer was obtained when viruses were coupled by the amino acid residues and their carbohydrate oxidized, or when viruses were coupled directly by their oxidized carbohydrate residues (Table 5).

Since these results were obtained with purified IgG preparations, it was necessary to determine whether the same correlation was valid for serum samples containing anti-CMV antibodies.

C. Determination of the Anti-CMV Antibody Titers of Sera from Healthy Donors by OCA ELISA, Adsorption ELISA, and Biological Neutralization

Sera were tested by OCA ELISA and adsorption ELISA, and the results obtained were compared with the neutralization antibody titer. The good correlation which was obtained with the IgG preparations was also obtained with serum samples from healthy individuals (Table 6).

D. OCA ELISA Titers of Sera from Patients with Ongoing CMV Infection

This suggested that the method developed could be applied directly to serum samples and as such was used to investigate the anti-CMV antibody titer of sera from patients with ongoing CMV infection. When this was done, no correlation was obtained between the OCA ELISA titers and the neutralization titers (Table 7).

Table 6 Titers of CMV Antibodies in Sera from Healthy Individuals

Serum sample no.	Adsorption ELISA titer[a]	Neutralization assay titer	Oxidized oligosaccharide attached ELISA titer[b]
1	6,400	160	125
2	26,600	320	250
3	102,400	640	2000
4	25,600	640	1000
5	102,400	2560	4000
6	25,600	2560	4000

[a]Correlation coefficient between neutralization assay titer and adsorption ELISA titer: +0.37.
[b]Correlation coefficient between neutralization assay titer and oxidized oligosaccharides attached ELISA titer: +0.96.

Among the reasons which were put forward for this lack of correlation was the existence in these sera of immunocomplexes formed between circulating CMV antigen and anti-CMV antibody. This was all the more probable since CMV antigens could be isolated from the urine of these patients.

We therefore undertook the development of experimental procedures which would permit the measurement of the specific anti-CMV titer in circulating immunocomplexes.

IV. IMMUNOCOMPLEXES

Present-day techniques for detecting immunocomplexes depend on the physico-chemical properties of these complexes or on their complement-binding activity. These procedures measure the amount of complexes present in sera regardless of their antigenic specificity but not the presence of complexes specific for particular antigens.

To overcome this problem our approach incorporated the fact that antigen-antibody complexes can be dissociated at an acid pH (2.3) and reassociated at an alkaline pH (8.1). If the reassociation is therefore performed in the presence of covalently immobilized antigen, then there should be competition between the covalently immobilized antigen and dissociated antigen for the dissociated antibody.

Table 7 Titers of CMV Antibodies in
Sera from Patients with Virus Present
in Urine

Neutralization titers	OCA ELISA titers
20	300
80	24,300
160	900
320	8,100
320	24,300
320	24,300
160	24,300
40	3,200
40	$>12,800$
40	$>12,800$
160	400
320	800
160	1,600
40	1,600
160	800
40	800
320	1,600
640	400
160	800
160	1,600

r=0.15

A. Verification of the Dissociation–Reassociation Procedure on the Reactivity of Free Antibody

To develop the procedure according to the theoretical considerations outlined above we first had to verify whether the acid treatment impaired the reactivity of free antibodies. This was verified experimentally using a hyperimmune rabbit serum antiparainfluenza virus (PIV). It is apparent (Fig. 12) that the dissociation and reassociation procedures had no effect on the free antibody titer.

B. Validation of the Dissociation and Reassociation Procedures for the Measurement of Antibody Titers in Experimentally Produced Immunocomplexes: PIV-Rabbit Anti-PIV

This rabbit serum was used for making experimental immunocomplexes by adding purified PIV virus to the antiserum, dissociating the complexes at pH

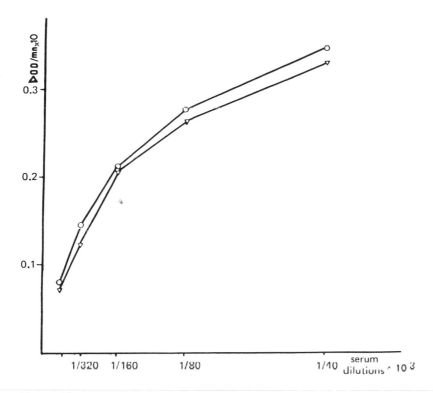

Figure 12   Rabbit serum containing parainfluenza virus (PIV) antibodies: (○) nondissociated; (△) dissociated and reassociated.

2.3, and reassociating the acid-treated serum at pH 8.1 *directly* in wells of a microtiter plate to which PIV was attached via its carbohydrate residues. It is apparent (Fig. 13) that the dissociation and reassociation procedure does permit the antibody present in the immunocomplexes to be measured. The appearance of a typical plate with site specifically coupled PIV and in which PIV anti-PIV immunocomplexes have been measured is shown in Figure 14.

C. Application of the Dissociation and Reassociation Procedure to Spermine-Antispermine Complexes Naturally Present in Human Serum

Verification of the efficiency of the acid dissociation and alkaline reassociation procedures was also carried out on the serum from a patient with bronchopulmonary cancer using the hapten spermine covalently bound to polyhydrazinostyrene microtiter plates. The results (Fig. 15) show that the free antispermine

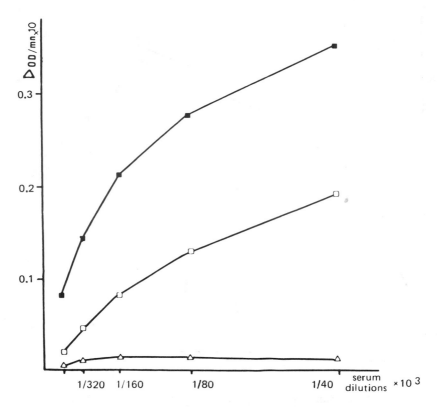

Figure 13 (■): Rabbit serum containing anti-PIV antibodies before adding PIV and nondissociated; (△): residual titer of free antibodies after adding PIV and nondissociated PIV; (□): titer of antibodies in immunocomplexes dissociation and reassociation. Rabbit IgG was measured by reaction with a goat serum anti-rabbit IgG labeled with alkaline phosphatase.

antibody titer of this serum is very low, whereas that of immunocomplex-bound antispermine antibodies is considerably higher.

D. Application of the Dissociation and Reassociation Procedure to the Serum from a Patient Before, During, and After CMV Infection

With the techniques validated, attempts were made to determine the titer of antibody in immunocomplexes present in the serum of a patient before, during, and after infection with CMV, by OCA ELISA. These OCA ELISA titers were compared to those obtained on adsorption ELISA. It is apparent (Table 8) that

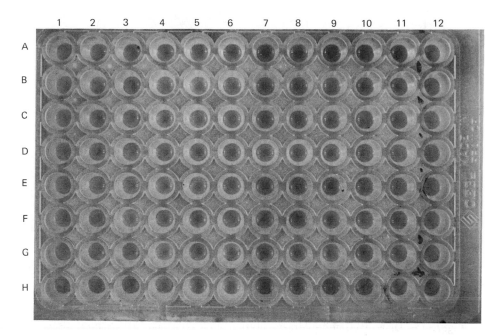

Figure 14 Substitution of the plate: Wells A to H in columns 1 to 6 contain no bound PIV. Wells A to H in columns 7 to 12 contain PIV (1 μg/well) bound covalently by carbohydrate residues. A rabbit serum anti-PIV was first diluted 1/100 in PBS, 0.1% Tween 20 and then incubated for 2 h at 37°C with different concentrations of PIV. Rows A and H contain the diluted antiserum alone; Rows B and E, C and F, D and G contain the diluted antiserum preincubated, respectively, with 0.75, 7.5, and 75 mg PIV/1. Samples at dilution of: Columns 1 and 7: 1/40,000; columns 2 and 8: 1/80,000; columns 3 and 9: 1/160,000; columns 4 and 10: 1/320,000; columns 5 and 11: 1/640,000. Columns 6 and 12: conjugate alone.

in the serum sample obtained *before* infection there is no difference between the adsorption ELISA titer and the OCA ELISA titer of free antibody (pH 8.1) or after dissociation and reassociation (pH 2.3 and pH 8.1). With the serum sample obtained from this patient at the time of active CMV infection (CMV present in the urine) the adsorption ELISA is greater than 12,800. The free antibody titer on OCA ELISA is less than 100 and the antibody titer in the immunocomplex is greater than 1,600. During convalescence when CMV is no longer present in urine the adsorption ELISA titer remains constant at 12,800, whereas the OCA ELISA titer of free antibody rises and that of immunocomplex-bound antibody remains constant at > 1,600. These results show that:

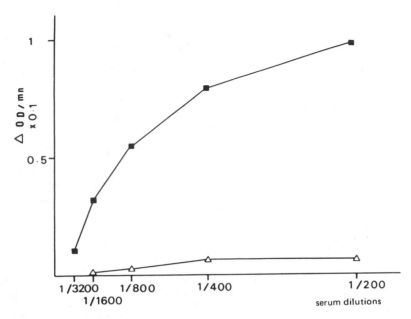

Figure 15 Diazotized polyhydrazidostyrene plates with covalently bound spermine were used to titer antispermine antibodies. Human Ig was measured by reaction with a goat serum anti-human Fc labeled with alkaline phosphatase.

Table 8 CMV Antibody Titers as Determined by Adsorption ELISA and OCA ELISA on Serial Serum Samples from the Same Patient

Date of sampling	Adsorption ELISA titer	O.C.A. ELISA titer		Virus in urine
		pH 8.1	pH 2.2 & pH 8.1	
2/17/85	100	100	100	0
6/27/85	≥12800	<100	≥1600	+
9/10/85	≥12800	>1600	≥1600	0

This serum was derived at the dates shown from the same patient suspected of having a CMV infection diagnosed by the presence of CMV in urine.

1. The adsorption ELISA titer does not vary with the clinical state whereas the OCA ELISA titer does fluctuate
2. When virus is present in urine, the immunocomplex-bound antibody titer, determined by OCA ELISA is greater than the free antibody titer
3. During convalescence when CMV was no longer present in urine there was a corresponding rise in the free antibody titer as measured by OCA ELISA.

These results could offer one explanation for the lack of correlation between OCA ELISA titers of free antibodies and neutralization antibody titers when samples were taken from patients with virus present in urine (Table 7).

V. DISCUSSION: ADVANTAGES AND FUTURE APPLICATIONS OF SITE SPECIFIC COUPLING

From the foregoing examples it should be apparent that the covalent coupling of antigens and antibodies is no longer a technology restricted to laboratories specialized in immunochemistry. Indeed, the availability of many different types of functionalized insoluble supports and also of homo- and heterobifunctional coupling agents permits site-specific covalent coupling of haptens, peptides, holoproteins, and glycoproteins to insoluble supports to be readily undertaken.

A. Supports

The choice of insoluble support is dependent on whether the test system to be developed is destined for quantitative or qualitative use in the field or in the laboratory.

For quantitative test systems such as agglutination with or without instrumentation, latex spheres are the obvious choice. When greater sensitivity is required an amplification step involving for example, some adaptation of an enzyme immunoassay (EIA) can be considered. The availability of magnetic and paramagnetic spheres (see Chap. 00 by Lau et al.) permits the passage from agglutination to EIA to be easily implemented.

For field tests or for regions with low technical infrastructure, there exists a choice between direct agglutination on one hand and EIA on magnetic spheres, on paramagnetic spheres, or on membranes in the form of "dip-sticks" on the other.

For laboratory assays, ELISA systems can be readily envisaged using polyhydrazido styrene plates as shown here, or other functionalized microtiter plates which are available commercially.

For qualitative assays, the latex spheres themselves can be used as markers in SEM (see Chap. 00 by Robert). When magnetizable particles are employed, they permit, in addition, the removal of unwanted cells from an heterogenous cell population such as tumor cells from bone marrow (see Chap. 00 by Combaret et al.) or of specific constituents such as protein-bound polyamines from plasma.

Site-specific coupling applied in this last context eliminates two potential problems: (a) loss of biological activity on coupling and (b) leakage from the insoluble support.This should permit the development of biocompatible devices capable of specifically eliminating high-molecular weight components from circulating blood (26).

B. Ligands

In the case of haptens their chemical heterogeneity is too extensive to enumerate all the different methods which can be applied. We have presented one example of an amine containing hapten putrescine bound by peptide bonds to carboxylated latex spheres. For other haptens the choice depends on the groups in the molecule which are involved in biological recognition, and those on which functionalities can be introduced for carrying out coupling procedures without affecting its functional integrity. Antibodies to nucleosides coupled to serum albumin via the ribose or base residues are a good example of this (27).

As regards peptides, these methods should find increased applications with the more increasingly widespread use of defined peptides for screening monoclonal antibodies. In this context it is well known that certain viral peptides, because of their size or low content of hydrophobic residues adsorb poorly or sometimes not at all to membranes (nitrocellulose, nylon) presently in use. This difficulty should be overcome by applying some of the methods described above to form amide bonds between carboxyl groups on the peptide and amine groups on the support or between diazotized acid hydrazide groups on the support and amine groups (N-terminal or ϵ NH$_2$ of lysines) on the peptide. Free sulfhydryl (SH) groups not implicated in biological activity of peptides are another obvious choice for site-specific immobilization using any one of a number of commercially available substituted iiodoacetamides or maleimides. The use of such SH-specific reagents for protein coupling has previously been demonstrated by several authors (28,29).

With holoproteins, the same site-specific coupling procedures used for peptides should be employed in screening monoclonal antibodies reactive with the native protein. We have had the unfortunate experience of selecting monoclonal antibodies which were reactive with an enzyme adsorbed to nitrocellulose, but which showed little or no interaction with the enzyme in its native state in solution. This observation provides yet another example of the distortion of antigenic sites which can take place on adsorption.

As regards the site-specific covalent coupling of glycoproteins, this aspect has been the main thrust of this review. We have provided evidence using viral glycoproteins derived from CMV that the antibody titers obtained on ELISA with amine-coupled CMV glycoproteins are greater than those found with carbo-hydrate-coupled CMV glycoproteins.

This difference in reactivity of amine-coupled and carbohydrate-coupled glycoproteins is not due to the coupling technique per se, but rather to the modification of carbohydrate residues during the oxidation step prior to coupling. This conclusion was drawn from the results presented in Table 4 in which CMV glycoproteins were first attached via their amine groups and then subsequently oxidized with periodate. Such amine-attached carbohydrate-oxidized virus gave results on ELISA which were identical to those obtained with oxidized carbohydrate-attached virus.

The importance of viral carbohydrate residues to the immune response had previously been documented for adenovirus 5 (25) where a similar periodate oxidation procedure employed on intact virions resulted in the loss of HA activity but not in the capacity to elicit neutralizing antibodies on the immunization of guinea pigs.

In this context can be placed our observations with CMV showing that there is a good correlation between Ab titers on OCA ELISA and the biological neutralization titers of IgG preparations. It is noteworthy that contrary to the observation made on OCA ELISA there was no correlation between titers obtained on NH₂ ELISA, or on adsorption ELISA and biological neutralization.

Our interpretation of the above results is as follows: antibody titers obtained with CMV attached via free amino groups on its protein moieties (NH₂ ELISA) represent the overall titers of antibodies reacting with both carbo-hydrates and proteins. On the contrary, the antibody titers obtained with amine-attached carbohydrate-oxidized virus or with oxidized carbohydrate-attached virus (OCA ELISA) are representative of antibodies reacting primarily with proteins.

At this stage of experimentation we must say "primarily with proteins" and not "uniquely with proteins" because we have not yet assessed whether oxidized virus still contains any remaining intact carbohydrates. What we do know however, is that oxidation of carbohydrates did take place, since aldehyde groups are generated on virus subjected to periodate treatment. On an average, oxidized PIV or CMV virus contained about 100 nmol equivalent glyceralde-hyde groups/mg proteins. Some of these aldehyde groups have been generated on glycoproteins since oxidized PIV treated with fluorescein acid hydrazide and separated on PAGE showed fluorescent protein bands. Whether this degree of oxidation was sufficient to perturb the antigenicity of *all* the carbohydrate moieties present on the virus is not known, but what can be said with certainty is that there was no further increase in aldehyde content on prolonging oxidation or on increasing the periodate concentration.

Interference by carbohydrate with the immune response has also been reported by other authors (30,31) who have shown quite clearly that deglycosylated viruses obtained after treatment with N-glycanase or with O-glycanase are better immunogens in terms of the neutralizing antibody response than viruses with intact carbohydrates.

These results from the literature provide additional justification for adopting site-specific covalent coupling when assaying antibody titers by ELISA in that this methodology, contrary to adsorption ELISA, permits at the very least, the quantification of antibodies with different specificities.

Finally the methodology as presently developed has permitted us to determine the titers of specific antibody present in circulating immunocomplexes (CIC). In the case of a patient with ongoing CMV infection it allowed us to clearly distinguish between the period of active infection and that of convalescence. This could not be achieved with adsorption ELISA.

But a further development which can be easily envisaged is the measurement of antigen present in CIC by immobilizing the corresponding antibody.

This could be of inestimable value in understanding syndromes related to the presence of circulating immunocomplexes in both infectious diseases and in autoimmune pathological states.

ACKNOWLEDGMENTS

Many colleagues have contributed over the years to various aspects of this work. We must thank in particular Dr. A. Niveleau for all the work done on Scanning electron microscopy. Dr. J. Grange and Mr. T. Keolouanghkot for their contributions to the nephelometric assays, and Dr. M. Aymard for her participation in the influenza assays.

We are also indebted to Dr. J. D. Rodwell (Cytogen Corporation) for stimulating discussions on OCA ELISA and to Drs. N. Kessler, M. P. Layani, and N. Pigat (Faculté de Médecine, Lyon) for samples of PIV virus and anti-PIV antiserum.

The technical assistance of Mr. G. Mollaret and Mme. M. F. Jacquier is gratefully acknowledged. The efficient secretarial help of Mme. A. Mary was an invaluable asset throughout these studies.

Financial support for this work was provided in part by "Agence Nationale pour la Valorisation de la Recherche" (ANVAR, Paris, France—contract No. A8206093) and Cytogen Corporation (Princeton, NJ, USA, contract No. 85.4783.00). V. Thomas and S. El Alaoui are the recipients of Cytogen fellowships.

REFERENCES

1. Fair, B. D., and Jamieson, A. M. (1980). Studies of protein adsorption on polystyrene latex surfaces. *J. Colloid Interface Sci. 77*:525–534.

2. Morrissey, B., and Han, C. C. (1978). The conformation of γ-globulin adsorbed on polystyrene latices determined by quasielastic light scattering. *J. Colloid Interface Sci.* 65:423–431.
3. Miller, J. V., Cuatrecasas, P., and Thomson, E. B. (1972). Purification of tyrosine aminotransferase by affinity chromatography. *Biochim. Biophys. Acta 276*:407–415.
4. Molday, R. S., Dreyer, W. J., Rembaum, A., and Yen, S. P. S. (1975). New immunolatex spheres. Visual markers of antigens on lymphocytes for scanning electron microscopy. *J. Cell Biol. 64*:75–88.
5. Avrameas, S. (1969). The cross-linking of proteins with glutaraldehyde and its use for the preparation of immunoadsorbants. *Immunochemistry 6*:53–65.
6. Monzan, P., Puzo, G., and Mazarguil, H. (1975). Etude du mécanisme d'établissement des liaisons glutaraldehyde-proteines. *Biochimie 57*:1281–1292.
7. Quash, G. (1979). Nouveaux tests d'agglutination pour la détection des virus de la grippe et réactifs pour la réalisation de ces tests. French Patent No. 2,450,877.
8. Cuatrecasas, P., and Anfinsen, C. B. (1971). Affinity chromatography. *Ann. Rev. Biochem. 40*:259–278.
9. Quash, G., Roch, A. M., Niveleau, A., Grange, J., Keolouangkhot, T., and Huppert, J. (1978). The preparation of latex particles with covalently bound polyamines, IgG and measles agglutinins and their use in visual agglutinations tests. *J. Immunol. Methods 22*:165–174.
10. O'Shannessy, D., and Quarles, R. H. (1987). Labeling of the oligosaccharide moieties of immunoglobulins. *J. Immunol. Methods 99*:153–161.
11. Rademacher, T. W., and Dwek, R. A. (1983). Structural, functional and conformational analysis of immunoglobulin G-derived asparagine-linked oligosaccharides. In *Progress in Immunology V*. Edited by Y. Yamamura and T. Tada, pp. 95–112, Academic Press, New York.
12. Aymard-Henry, M., Coleman, M. T., Dowdle, W. R., Laver, W. G., Schild, G. C., and Webster, R. G. (1973). Influenza virus neuraminidase and neuraminidase-inhibition test procedures. *Bull. World Health Org. 48*:199–202.
13. Warren, L. (1959). The thiobarbituric acid assay of sialic acids. *J. Biol. Chem. 234*:1971–1975.
14. Quash, G. A., Aymard, M., Fougerouze, J., and Ripoll, H. (1982). A fetuin-latex agglutination test for detecting the neuraminidases of myxoviruses in allantoic fluid. *J. Biol. Stand. 10*:115–124.
15. Aymard, M., Quash, G. A., and Million, J. (1982). Determination of anti-neuraminidase antibody titres in human sera by inhibition of the agglutination of fetuin-latex by influenza viruses. *J. Biol. Stand. 10*:125–133.
16. Ripoll, J. P., Roch, A. M., Quash, G. A., and Grange, J. (1980). An automatic continuous flow method for the determination of antipolyamine antibodies in human sera. *J. Immunol. Methods 33*:159–173.

17. Israel, A., Niveleau, A., Quash, G., and Richard, M. H. (1979). Latex fetuin spheres as probes for influenza virus neuraminidase in productively and abortively infected cells. *Arch. Virol. 61*:183–199.
18. Quash, G. A., Niveleau, A., Aupoix, M., and Greenland, T. (1976). Immunolatex visualisation of cell surface Forssman and polyamine antigens. *Exp. Cell Res. 98*:253–261.
19. Treleaven, J. G., Ugelstad, J., Philip, T., Gibson, F. M., Rembaum, A., and Caine, G. D. (1984). Removal of neuroblastoma cells from bone marrow with monoclonal antibodies conjugated to magnetic microspheres. *Lancet 14*:70–73.
20. Molday, R. S., Yen, S. P. S., and Rembaum, A. (1977). Application of magnetic microspheres in labelling and separation of cells. *Nature 68*:437–438.
21. Roch, A. M., Quash, G. A., Ripoll, H., Vigreux, B., and Niveleau, A. (1981). In *Advances in Polyamine Research*. Edited by C. M. Caldarera, V. Zappia, and U. Bachrach, Raven Press, New York, pp. 225–235.
22. Delcros, J. G., Roch, A. M., Thomas, V., El Alaoui, S., Moulinoux, J. P., and Quash, G. (1987). Protein-bound polyamines in the plasma of mice grafted with the Lewis lung carcinoma. *FEBS Lett. 220*:236–242.
23. Chin, N. W., and Links, K. W. (1977). Covalent attachment of lactoperoxidase to polystyrene tissue culture flasks. *Anal. Biochem. 83*:709–719.
24. Quash, G. A. (1985). Nouveaux reactifs de diagnostic. French Patent No. 85,17,377.
25. Dreesman, G. R., and Suriano, J. R. (1976). Alteration of adenovirus antigenic sites and infectivity by periodate oxidation. *Virology 69*:700–709.
26. Virella, G., and Glassman, A. B. (1986). Apheresis, exchange, adsorption and filtration of plasma: Four approaches to the removal of undesirable circulating substances. *Biomed. Pharmacother. 40*:286–296.
27. Sela, M., and Fuchs, S. (1967). Preparation of nucleoside conjugates of synthetic polypeptides. In *Methods in Immunology and Immunochemistry*. Edited by C. A. Williams and M. W. Chase, pp. 185–186, Academic Press, New York and London.
28. Bernatowicz, M. S., and Matsueda, G. R. (1985). The N-hydroxysuccinimide ester of BOC-(S-(3-nitro-2-pyridine-sulfenyl)-cysteine: A heterobifunctional cross-linking agent. *Biochem. Biophys. Res. Commun. 132*:1046–1050.
29. Yoshitake, S., Yamada, Y., Ishikawa, E., and Masseyef, R. (1979). Conjugation of glucose oxidase from Aspergillus niger and rabbit antibodies using N-hydroxysuccinimide ester of N-(-4-carboxycyclohexylmethyl)-maleimide. *Eur. J. Biochem. 101*:395–399.
30. Elder, J. H., and Alexander, S. (1982). Endo-β-N-acetylglucosaminidase F: endoglycosidase from *Flavobacterium meningosepticum* that cleaves both high-mannose and complex glycoproteins. *Proc. Natl. Acad. Sci. USA 79*: 4540–4544.
31. Montelaro, R. C., West, M., and Issel, C. J. (1984). Antigenic reactivity of the major glycoprotein of equine infectious anemia virus, a retrovirus. *Virology 136*:368–374.

9

A Highly Sensitive EIA Utilizing Covalent Conjugate of a Polymerized Enzyme and an Antibody

SUSAN Y. TSENG, J. WILLIAM FREYTAG, and ALAN R. CRAIG
E. I. du Pont de Nemours & Co., Inc., Wilmington, Delaware

I. INTRODUCTION

The use of enzyme-labeled antibodies in immunochemical detection was first reported in 1966 by Avrameas and Uriel (1) and Nakane and Kawaoi (2). However, the important contribution that these reagents would make to diagnostic medicine was not recognized until 1971, when Engvall and Perlmann (3) and Van Weeman and Schuurs (4) described the use of antibody–enzyme conjugates in quantitative enzyme-linked immunoassays. Since that time, numerous procedures for coupling antibodies or antibody fragments to various enzymes have been developed.

Enzyme immunometric assays (EIAs) are a class of heterogeneous immunoassays that have achieved widespread use in diagnostic medicine. Each of these assays employs a specific enzyme-labeled antibody, which is mixed with a sample containing the target analyte. After a brief incubation period to allow antibody and analyte to bind, the excess unreacted antibody-enzyme conjugate is removed. The enzyme in this antigen-bound fraction produces a signal that can be quantified and used to directly measure the analyte concentration in the sample.

Enzyme immunometric assays are divided into two types, based on the configuration of the target analyte: one-site assays are used with analytes possessing only a single antigenic determinant; two-site, or "sandwich," assays are used with analytes that have two or more different antigenic determinants or a single, multiply occurring determinant.

One of the most important factors governing the ultimate usefulness of an EIA is the nature and quality of the antibody–enzyme conjugate. To measure analytes of very low concentration, a conjugate with a strong signal amplifier is required. It has been appreciated for some time that signal generation in EIA can be greatly enhanced if polymeric antibody–enzyme conjugates are substituted for monomeric conjugates.

Originally, aggregated antibody–enzyme conjugates were produced using a nonspecific coupling chemistry such as glutaraldehyde crosslinking (5) or a periodate oxidation method (6). Unfortunately, when nonspecific coupling reactions are used to prepare conjugates, crosslinking is random and the antibodies, or antibody fragments, are often buried deep within the aggregated complex—thus remaining largely inaccessible for antigen binding. In addition, these amorphous macromolecular complexes are difficult to prepare in a reproducible fashion and they routinely suffer from very high background blanks (due to nonspecific binding), which dramatically reduces the sensitivity that can be achieved with the corresponding assays (7).

More recently, several procedures were described that used noncovalent interactions to generate conjugates with high enzyme-to-antibody ratios. Such conjugates were prepared for: peroxidase/antiperoxidase and phosphatase/antiphosphatase (8); protein A–peroxidase conjugate/antiprotein A-peroxidase conjugates (9); biotin-labeled antibody and peroxidase–avidin complexes (10); and antibody-labeled bovine serum albumin (BSA) and enzyme-labeled anti-BSA (11). Although these procedures do generally provide enhanced signals, they all suffered from the limitations of reversible binding phenomena, such as unwanted dissociation and affinity limitations. A reproducible method for preparing well-defined covalently linked polymeric enzyme–antibody conjugates was needed.

This report describes the preparation and evaluation of two such conjugates: Fab'-β-galactosidase and IgG-horseradish peroxidase (HRP). In both cases, the enzyme was prepolymerized in a controlled fashion before it was coupled to the antibody or antibody fragment. β-galactosidase, which contains 20–40 free–SH groups per molecule, can be polymerized directly. HRP, however, has fewer than two primary amine groups per molecule, so direct polymerization is difficult. This problem was overcome by attaching multiple copies of HRP to an activated polymer backbone of polyacrylic acid (PAA).

II. PREPARATION OF THE Fab'-β-GALACTOSIDASE CONJUGATE

To prepare the Fab'-β-galactosidase conjugate, β-galactosidase was prepolymerized by dissolving it to a concentration of 4 mg/ml in a solution of 50mM phosphate, 0.15M NaCl, 0.001M MgCl$_2$, and 0.002M EDTA at pH 7.5. The enzyme solution was then treated with various amounts of o-phenylenedimaleimide (O-PDM) that had been freshly dissolved in N,N'-dimethylformamide at a concentration of 3.7 mM. After 1 hour at 4°C, the reaction was terminated by adding 10 μl of 0.1M 2-mercaptoethylamine solution, followed by a 30-min incubation period at room temperature. A small aliquot of the enzyme solution was tested for β-galactosidase activity, and the rest of the solution was subjected to gel filtration on a Sepharose 6B-CL column (1.0 X 45 cm) equilibrated in phosphate-NaCl-MgCl$_2$ buffer (no EDTA). After chromatography, the column effluent was also tested for β-galactosidase activity.

The resulting polymeric enzyme sizes were analyzed by gel filtration on Sephacryl S-1000 resin, which has a fractionation range of 125 Å to greater than 2000 Å Stokes' radius. Figure 1 shows the calibration curve of an S-1000 column developed in neutral aqueous solution using standard polystyrene spheres (Dow Chemical polystyrene standards) as size markers (12). This resin was found to be quite useful for approximating the molecular size of the polymerized enzyme complexes. The molecular weights of the complexes were calculated from the Stokes' radius (assuming a spherical shape and a partial specific volume of 0.75 cm^3/g for the protein).

The Fab' portion of the conjugate was prepared from digoxin-specific IgG. The IgG was immunopurified from rabbit antiserum in a one-step affinity chromatography procedure on a ouabain-BSA-agarose (ouabain is a digoxin analog) column (13). After purification, the digoxin-specific IgG was 95% pure, and was converted into F(ab')$_2$ fragments by pepsin digestion followed by filtration on a Sephadex G-150 column. The Fab'-SH fragments were generated from the F(ab')$_2$ by reducing the inter-heavy chain disulfides with 1mM 2-mercaptoethanol for 90 min at room temperature followed by desalting on Sephadex G-15 in 0.015M sodium phosphate, 0.15M NaCl, and 0.001M EDTA at pH 6.0.

The poly-β-galactosidase was then suspended in 0.05M sodium phosphate, 0.15M NaCl, 0.001M MgCl$_2$, and 0.002M EDTA at pH 6.5 and treated with a 50-molar excess of o-phenylenediamaleimide (dissolved at 10 mg/ml in N,N'-dimethylformamide) for a second time. After a 1-h reaction period at 25°C, the enzyme mixture was applied to a Sephadex G-25 column (1.5 X 30 cm) equilibrated with the same phosphate-NaCl–MgCl$_2$ buffer (no EDTA). The polymerized β-galactosidase-maleimide, which eluted in the void volume of the column, was collected and combined with various amounts of the freshly reduced affinity-purified antidigoxin Fab'-SH fragments.

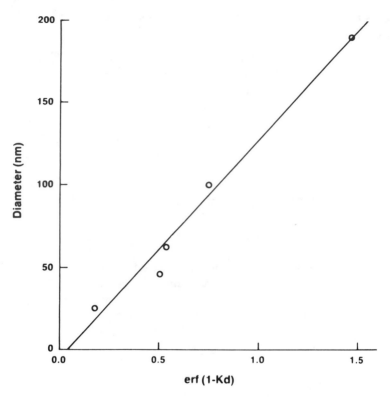

Figure 1 Calibration curve of Sephacryl S-1000 (1.0 × 45 cm) using standard polystyrene spheres. Data is plotted as the error function of the partition distribution (kD) versus the diameter of the polystyrene spheres. This calibration curve was used to estimate the molecular size of the polymerized β-galactosidase aggregates.

The conjugation of Fab'-SH plus maleimido-β-galactosidase was allowed to proceed at 25°C for 1 hour, and then subjected to column chromatography on a Sephacryl S-1000 column.

III. PREPARATION OF THE IgG-HRP CONJUGATE

To prepare the IgG-HRP conjugate, lyophilized horseradish peroxidase (HRP) was prepolymerized by dissolving it in polyacrylic acid (PAA) of a desired length (size range from 50,000–250,000 MW) in 0.1M sodium acetate buffer at pH 5.5. A 50-fold molar excess of solid 1-ethyl-3-(3'-dimethylaminopropyl) carbodimide, hydrochloride (EDCI) was then added directly to the solution.

After a 1-h reaction period at 25°C, an excess of glycine was added to the mixture to block the unreacted EDCI. The reaction mixture was then incubated at 25°C for an additional 30 minutes and subjected to gel filtration on a Sepharose CL-6B column (1.0 × 90 cm) using 0.1M acetate buffer at pH 5.5. The different fractions of polymeric HRP-PAA that eluted from the column were analyzed on a Du Pont HPLC Bio Series GF-250 column to determine their average size.

The polymeric HRP-PAA (1 × 10^6 daltons) was chosen and then mixed with IgG at ratios of 20/1 and 40/1 HRP/IgG (depending on the assay). To conjugate the IgG and the poly-HRP, EDCI was added directly to the mixture at a molar ratio of 50/1 EDCI/IgG. After a 1-h reaction period at 25°C, the various conjugates were purified on a Du Pont HPLC GF-250 XL column (21.5 mm × 25 cm) and eluted at a flow rate of 2 ml/min with citrate-NaCl-CaCl$_2$ buffer at pH 6.5.

IV. DISCUSSION

A method was needed to prepare well-defined covalently linked polymeric enzyme–antibody conjugates. This method had to: (1) be reproducible; (2) ensure that the antibodies or antibody fragments would be attached to the outside of the polymeric enzyme complex; and (3) ensure that the enzyme would not lose its activity after polymerization.

Two enzymes, β-galactosidase and horseradish peroxidase (HRP), were chosen to investigate the feasibility of such a method. After these enzymes were polymerized and coupled with antibody, the sensitivity of the resulting conjugates was analyzed in one-site and two-site (sandwich) immunometric assays.

β-Galactosidase was chosen for two reasons: (1) its insensitivity to potentially interfering substances that are present in most human biological specimens; and (2) the existence of multiple sulfhydryl residues that are not critical to the expression of full enzymatic activity. β-Galactosidase was polymerized (via a limited number of these sulfhydryl groups) with o-phenylenedimaleimide (O-PDM), a sulfhydryl-specific homobifunctional crosslinking reagent. It was found that the enzyme could be reproducibly polymerized in a controlled fashion to almost any size between 13 and 714 millions MW with only a minimal loss (< 15%) of enzymatic activity.

Several parameters control the degree of enzyme polymerization. One of the key factors is the molar ratio of O-PDM/β-galactosidase. Polymer size increases as the O-PDM/β-gal molar ratio increases (Fig. 2). The use of a fivefold molar excess of O-PDM caused greater than 50% of the original β-galactosidase to be crosslinked into a molecular aggregate of 20 million daltons or greater. A tenfold molar excess of O-PDM produced quantitative polymerization of the β-galactosidase into a very large enzyme complex. However, when a 200-fold excess of O-PDM was used, all sulfhydryl function groups were modified instantly and no crosslinking occurred.

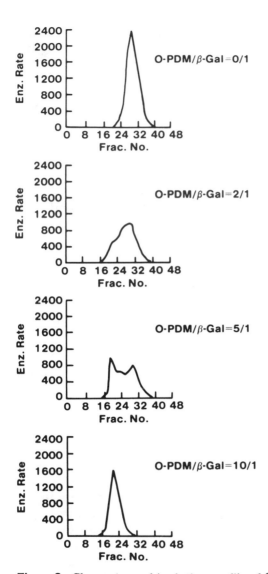

Figure 2 Chromatographic elution profile of β-galactosidase aggregates after polymerization with various amounts (0, 2, 5, and 10-fold molar excess) of o-phenylenediamaleimide. All samples were chromatographed on identical Sepharose 6B-CL columns (1.0 × 4.5 cm) equilibrated in phosphate-NaCl-MgCl₂ buffer, pH 7.5.

Table 1 Molecular Weight and Specific Activity of Polymerized β-Galactosidase as a Function of the Concentration of Enzyme Used in the Synthesis

[β-Galactosidase] (mg/ml)	Molec. wgt. (million)	Specific activity (μmol/min/mg)
4	714–870	562±4
3	39–66	603±6
2	16–20	529±4
1	3–4	530±4
Monomer	0.6	639±3

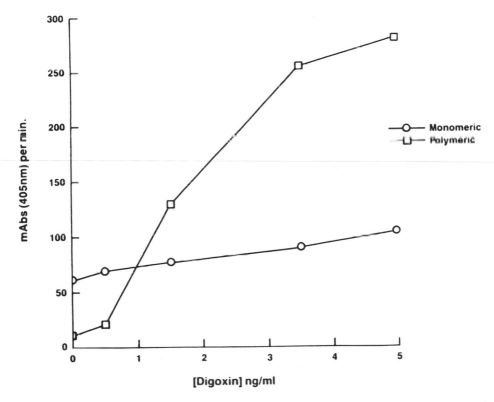

Figure 3 Standard calibration curves for monomeric versus polymeric β-galactosidase-Fab′ conjugates in an affinity column-mediated immunometric assay for digoxin. β-galactosidase activity in the unbound fraction (measured as the change in milliabsorbance units at 405 nm per minute) is plotted against the digoxin concentration in the original serum calibrator.

Another key parameter is the concentration of β-galactosidase. It was previously known that polymer size would increase proportionally with protein concentration, but the degree to which polymer size *depended* on protein concentration was completely unexpected. By changing the β-galactosidase concentration from 1 to 4 mg/ml (1.9 mM to 7.4 mM), the molecular size of the polymeric enzyme increased 200-fold, from 3.4×10^6 daltons to 8×10^8 daltons (Table 1). If polymerization is carried out at a protein concentration of 2 mg/ml and the O-PDM/β-galactosidase ratio is 5/1, the reaction will be complete after 1 hour. The resulting polymeric enzyme will contain, on the average, 65 molecules of β-galactosidase and will retain > 80% of its original enzyme activity.

After polymerization, O-PDM was used to covalently attach the monovalent Fab'−SH antibody fragments to the outside of the enzyme complex. Fab'−SH fragments were chosen because, by using the hinge region thiol group, covalent coupling could occur away from the antigen binding site. It was found that removal of the Fc portion of the antibody reduces nonspecific binding on solid surfaces (14).

The performance of the poly-β-gal-Fab' conjugate in an immunometric assay was then evaluated. An affinity column mediated immunoassay (ACMIA) for digoxin was chosen for this purpose.

The antibody–enzyme conjugate that performed best was a 35 million MW aggregate. The background activity of this conjugate was roughly equivalent to that of monomeric Fab'-β-galactosidase, but the conjugate exhibited a 10-fold enhancement in sensitivity (Fig. 3).

In this assay, an excess,but optimal amount of the conjugate was first mixed with the analyte (digoxin) and allowed to react for 30 min. The mixture was then passed through an antigen affinity column at a controlled rate. The eluent, which contains only analyte that reacted with the conjugate, was collected and

Table 2 Sensitivity and Background in Digoxin Affinity Column-Mediated Immunometric Assay with Various Size of Conjugates

Conjugate MWT (million)	Background (mAbs/min)	Slope sensitivity (mAbs/min/ng/ml)
714	378	308
35	75	108
20	101	35
13	44	25
0.6	20	10

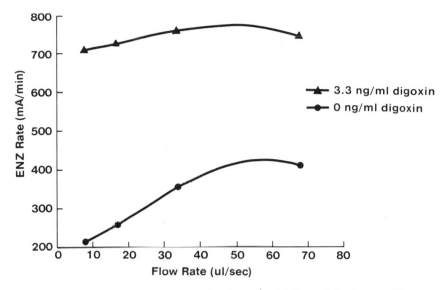

Figure 4   Effect of elution rate on the slope sensitivity and background in an affinity column-mediated immunometric assay for digoxin. (▲-▲) 3.3 mg/ml digoxin, (●-●) 0 mg/ml digoxin in serum calibrator. β-galactosidase activity in the unbound fraction (measured as the change in milliabsorbance units at 405 nm/min) is plotted against affinity column flow rate.

Table 3   Sensitivity and Background in Digoxin Affinity Column Mediated Immunometric Assay with Various Conjugates of Same Size But Different Number of Antigen-Binding Sites Per Molecule

Ab-ENZ conjugate	B-Gal/Fab' molar/ratio	Background (mAbs/min)	Slope sensitivity (mAbs/min/ng/ml)
1	1:8.8	0	0
2	1:3	0	12
3	1:1	39	37
4	1:0.5	77	68
5	1:0.25	1054	267

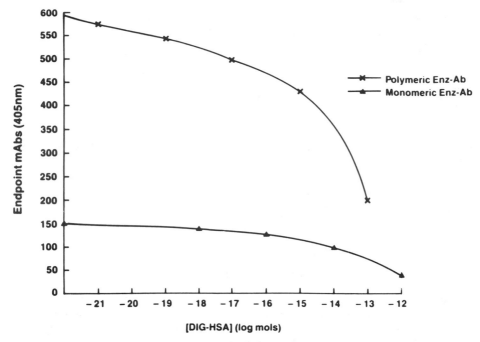

Figure 5 Standard calibration curves for monomeric versus polymeric β-galac-tosidase-Fab′ conjugates in an antibody affinity column-mediated immuno-metric assay for digoxin-HSA two-site sandwich EIA. β-galactosidase activity in the unbound fraction (measured as milliabsorbance units at 405 nm) is plotted against the digoxin-HSA concentration in the PBS/BSA buffer calibrator.

reacted with substrate to quantitate the amount of conjugate-analyte complex that was present. The signal gathered in this manner is directly proportional to the analyte concentration in the original sample.

In the ACMIA for digoxin, the poly-β-gal-Fab′ conjugate can provide 20–30 times more signal than the monomeric conjugate. The polymeric conjugate permits the quantitation of as little as $10^{-11} M$ analyte in a 40-min assay.

It was found that two factors affect the sensitivity of the poly-β-gal-Fab′ conjugate in ACMIA: (1) size and (2) number of antibody binding sites per conjugate molecule. Assay slope sensitivity is directly proportional to enzyme polymer size; the larger the conjugate molecule, the greater the sensitivity (Table 2). Although background also increases in proportion to conjugate size, it was found that if the flow rate of the affinity column is decreased when a large conjugate is used, background will drop dramatically (Fig. 4).

In ACMIA, the number of antibody binding sites per conjugate affects slope sensitivity inversely; as the number of binding sites increases, the assay becomes less sensitive and the background decreases (Table 3).

The sensitivity of the poly-β-gal-Fab' conjugate for digoxin was also evaluated in a two-site (sandwich) enzyme immunoassay. In sandwich assays, one antibody, which is attached to a solid support, captures the analyte; a second antibody, which is part of an antibody-enzyme conjugate, is then used to detect the analyte. Because it must bind at least two antibodies, any analyte used in a sandwich assay must be multivalent. Digoxin, which is monovalent, was turned into a synthetic multivalent hapten by coupling five digoxin molecules to a human serum albumin (HSA) molecule (13).

In the digoxin–HSA sandwich assay, the conjugate was incubated with various levels of digoxin–HSA for 60 min at room temperature. Only the antibody-enzyme conjugate that had not complexed with the antigen was passing through an antibody column. A fraction of this unbound conjugate was then quantified for enzymatic activity to indirectly determine the analyte level. It was found

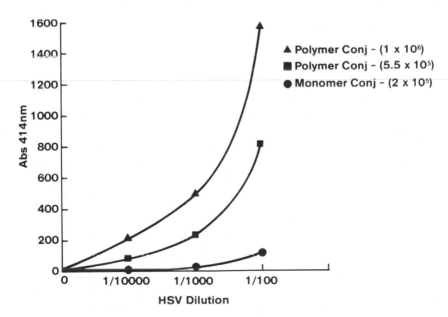

Figure 6 Standard calibration curve for monomeric versus polymeric HRP-anti-HSV1 IgG conjugates in a HSV1 two-site sandwich EIA. HRP activity in the bound fraction (measured as milliabsorbance units at 414 nm) is plotted against the HSV1 viral lysate dilutions.

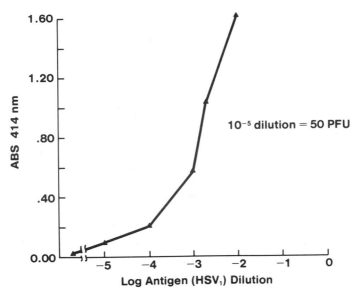

Figure 7 Standard calibration curve for a polymeric HRP-anti-HSV1-IgG conjugate (1.3×10^6 M.WT.) in HSV1 sandwich EIA. HRP activity in the bound fraction (measured as milliabsorbance units at 414 nm) is plotted against the HSV1 viral lysate dilution in PBS/BSA buffer calibrator.

that the polymeric conjugate could detect as little as 1×10^{-21} mol of digoxin-HSA (equivalent to $1 \times 10^{-16} M$ digoxin), indicating a degree of sensitivity 10^4 times greater than that possible with the corresponding monomeric reference conjugate (Fig. 5).

Horseradish peroxidase (HRP) is difficult to polymerize directly, because it has fewer than two primary amine groups per molecule. This problem was overcome by attaching multiple copies of HRP to an polymer backbone of polyacrylic acid (PAA) that had first been activated with 1-ethyl-3-(3'-dimethylaminopropyl) carbodimide hydrochloride (EDCI). As with poly-β-galactosidase, the poly-HRP-PAA was affected by both the molar ratios of the reactants (EDCI/PAA and HRP/PAA) and the protein concentration.

After multiple copies of HRP were attached to the PAA backbone, the polyenzyme was chemically crosslinked with antibody to create a poly–HPR–Ab conjugate. A model system was created in which the polyenzyme was attached to antiherpes simplex virus I (HSV I) antibody and used in a HSV I sandwich assay. Figure 6 compares the sensitivity of different sizes of poly-HRP-anti-HSV I-IgG. It was found that the poly-HRP-anti-HSV-Ab conjugate could detect a 1/500,000 dilution of HSV I viral lysate, which is equivalent to 50 PFU of HSV I (Fig. 7).

V. CONCLUSIONS

By controlling the size of the polyenzyme, the number of antibody binding sites, and the flow rate of the affinity column, a method for consistently preparing well-defined covalently linked polymeric enzyme-antibody conjugates was successfully developed. These polyenzyme–antibody conjugates were sensitive enough to detect analyte concentrations of $10^{-11}M$ in one-site and $10^{-16}M$ in two-site sandwich enzyme immunometric assays. If a fluorogenic substrate was used, this sensitivity could be enhanced 50-100-fold.

REFERENCES

1. Avrameas, S., and Uriel, J. (1966). Method of antigen and antibody labeling with enzymes and its immunodiffusion application. *C. R. Seances Acad. Sci. Ser. D 262*:2543–2545.
2. Nakane, P. K., and Kawaoi, A. (1974). Peroxidase-labeled antibody. A new method of conjugation. *J. Histochem. Cytochem. 22*:1084–1091.
3. Engvall, E. P., and Perlmann, P. (1971). Enzyme-linked immunosorbent assay (ELISA). Quantitative assay of immunoglobulin G. *Immunochemistry 8*:871–874.
4. Van Weeman, B. K., and Schuurs, A. H. W. M. (1971). Immunoassay using antigen-enzyme conjugate. *FEBS Letters 15*:232–236.
5. Engvall, E. P. (1978). Preparation of enzyme-labeled *Staphylococcal* protein A and its use for detection of antibodies. *Scand. J. Immunol. 8*(suppl. 7): 25–31.
6. Boorsma, D. M., and Streefkerk, J. G. (1979). Periodate or glutaraldehyde for preparing peroxidase conjugate. *J. Immunol. Method 30*:245–255.
7. Ishikawa, E. M., et al. (1982). Major factors limiting sensitivity of sandwich enzyme immunoassay for ferritin; immunoglobulin E, and thyroid-stimulating hormone. *Ann. Clin. Biochem. 19*:379–384.
8. Hessian, P. A., Highton, J., and Palmer, D. G. (1986). Development of an enzyme immunoassay for the quantitation of cellular antigen expression. *J. Immunol. Methods 91*:29–34.
9. Holbeck, S. L., and Nepom, G. T. (1983). Enhanced detection of immunoglobulin binding by a modified ELISA. *J. Immunol. Methods 60*:47–52.
10. Yolken, R. H., et al. (1983). Enzyme immunoassays for the detection of bacterial antigens utilizing biotin-labeled antibody and peroxidase biotin-abidin complex. *J. Immunol. Methods 56*:319–327.
11. Guesdon, J. L., et al. (1983). An amplification system using BSA-antibody conjugate for sensitive enzyme immunoassay. *J. Immunol. Methods 58*: 133–142.
12. Nozaki, Y., et al. (1982). Size analysis of phospholipid vesicle preparations. *Science 217*:366–367.
13. Freytag, J. W., et al. (1984). A highly sensitive Affinity-Column-Mediated Immunometric Assay, as exemplified by digoxin. *Clin. Chem. 30*:417–420.

14. Ishikawa, E. M., et al. (1983). Enzyme-labeling of antibodies and their fragments for enzyme immunoassay and immunohistochemical staining. *J. Immunoassay* 4:209–327.

10

Immobilization of Antigens and Antibodies on Chromium Dioxide Magnetic Particles for Use in Immunodiagnostic Assays

H. PHILLIP LAU, ROBIN RESCH CHARLTON, ESTHER K. YANG, AND WARREN K. MILLER

E. I. du Pont de Nemours & Co., Inc., Glasgow Research Laboratory, Wilmington, Delaware

I. INTRODUCTION

Immunoassays for the measurement of hormones, cancer markers and infectious disease markers usually use microtiter plates or polystyrene beads as the solid support. Although these assays generally offer adequate sensitivity and specificity, they take a long time to complete, typically 4 to 24 h. Much of this time is required to capture the analytes on the solid support. Thus, the choice of solid support is the key to the speed of solid phase immunoassays.

We have developed a new magnetic particle solid support for use in immunodiagnostic assays. The magnetic, physical, and stability properties of magnetic tape chromium dioxide (CrO_2) particles have been significantly altered to provide a stable, aqueous slurry to which antigen and antibody can be attached. Several covalent linkages and passive adsorption approaches have been investigated and the use of a glutaraldehyde-activated amino group is the preferred method of coupling protein to the particles.

Previous authors have discussed the advantages of magnetic particles as a solid support in immunoassays, for example magnetizable charcoal (1) or

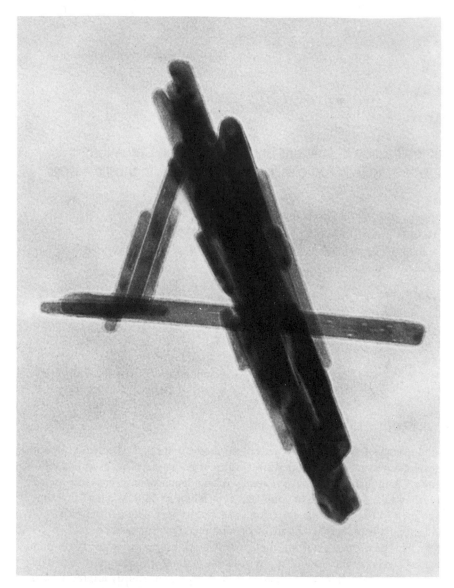

Figure 1 Electron micrograph of stabilized chromium dioxide particles.

paramagnetic ferrous oxide particles (2). General advantages of magnetic particle solid supports are that: particles offer high surface area which enhances capture capacity; particles suspended in solution reduce the diffusion time of the species to be captured, thus shortening the assay time. Magnetic separation is also efficient and easy to handle. It does not require cumbersome centrifugation or filtration steps, and is amenable to automation. In addition, the chromium dioxide magnetic particles we developed (3,4) are hydrophilic and readily dispersed. They are very stable in aqueous suspension and the surface can be functionalized for covalent binding of antigens or antibodies.

The chromium dioxide magnetic particle technology stems from Du Pont's extensive experience in the development and manufacture of chromium dioxide particles for magnetic recording. However, the desirable properties for magnetic recording are significantly different from those needed for an ideal solid support to be used in diagnostic assays. We have developed a multistep coating process to create particles suitable for immunoassay applications. This technology, coupled with Du Pont's expanding biotechnology capabilities for developing monoclonal antibodies and conjugates, has supplied the foundation for our development of novel magnetic particle-based immunoassays.

The particles are ferromagnetic but have low remanent magnetism, thus allowing rapid separation and resuspension for incubation, washing, and measurement steps. The high surface area (> 40 m^2/g) provides very rapid immunochemical capture and very short assay time. Thus when the particles are coupled to antibodies with high affinity and specificity, immunoassays for low-level hormones, cancer markers, and infectious disease agents can be performed very rapidly with state-of-the-art performance. The particles have also been coupled to antigen for immunoassay of low-level drugs, vitamins, and steroid hormones.

The particle size, surface area, and protein uptake capacity of the assay quality particles have been specifically designed for optimal assay performance and product utility. As you can see in the electron micrograph (Fig. 1), chromium dioxide particles are needle-shaped and nonporous. The specific surface area is 40 m^2/g, agglomerate size ranges from 2 to 5 microns, and protein uptake capacity is up to 40 mg/g particles. This loading capacity is many times greater than commonly used beads.

Magnetic tape chromium dioxide particles have poor hydrolytic stability and are not acceptable for use in immunoassays. Resolving this instability was a key challenge in the development of the diagnostic particles. Insight into understanding the instability mechanism in concert with Du Pont's expertise, has produced particles which exhibit no measurable instability. When antigens or antibodies are covalently attached to them, the resulting reagents are stable for longer than 6 months at 4°C.

This long-term hydrolytic stability along with desirable dispersion properties are achieved by a three-step coating process as described in Figure 2. The

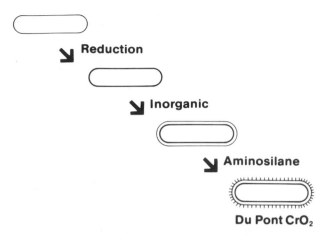

Figure 2 Process of chromium dioxide magnetic particle stabilization.

chromium dioxide surface is first reduced under controlled conditions to generate a nonreactive layer. The reduced surface is then totally encapsulated with an inorganic material to prevent reoxidation. Finally, the surface is coated with a common organosilane to provide various functional groups for protein attachment. This process retains the strong magnetic properties of chromium dioxide for rapid separation but converts them to particles that can be resuspended easily. It also allows efficient washing which minimizes nonspecific binding and matrix effects. These are the key advantages of chromium dioxide particles over other magnetic particles.

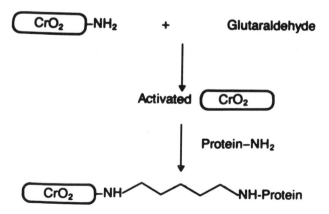

Figure 3 Coupling of protein to chromium dioxide particles.

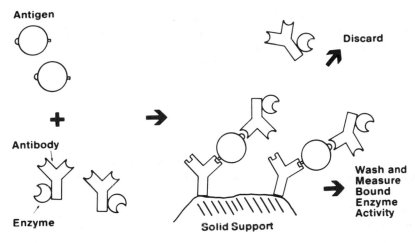

Figure 4 Immobilized antibodies in two-site sandwich solid-phase enzyme immunoassay.

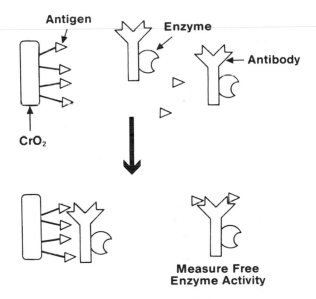

Figure 5 Immobilized antigens in immunoenzymometric assay.

Immobilization of antigens and antibodies on the coated chromium dioxide particles can be achieved by various common protein immobilization techniques. We have tried adsorption on chloromethyl phenyl silane-coated particles, carbodiimide coupling on carboxylic acid surface, direct attachment on epoxy surface, and many other protein immobilization techniques. In our experience, the best performance was achieved by coupling the protein to glutaraldehyde-activated aminosilane-coated particles as shown in Figure 3. We will limit our discussion to the aminosilane-coated particles and the glutaraldehyde activation protein immobilization method.

Antibodies selected for high affinity and specificity are attached to the chromium dioxide particles and are used on both one-site competitive binding and two-site immunometric approaches. The two-site approach (Fig. 4) is intended to measure large molecules with multiple binding sites, for example, follitropin follicle-stimulating hormone, FSH) and markers of infectious disease. In this case, the sample is incubated, either sequentially or simultaneously, with antibody attached to chromium dioxide particles and with a second, labeled antibody. During the incubation period, the first antibody captures the analyte and binds it to the chromium dioxide particles, while the second antibody binds to the captured analyte, thus labeling it. Following incubation, the particles are separated magnetically and washed to remove excess antibody and serum interferences. The label on the particles is quantified and is directly proportional to the analyte concentration in the original sample.

Antigens can also be attached to the chromium dioxide particles directly or through a spacer arm and used in both immunometric competitive or immunoenzymometric assays (5). The immunoenzymometric approach, which can be used to measure both large and small molecules (for example, β-human chorionic gonadotropin and digoxin), is shown diagrammatically in Figure 5. β-galactosidase antibody conjugate is incubated with the sample. During the incubation period, analyte in the sample binds to the antibody. Following incubation, chromium dioxide particles containing the analyte or analyte analog are added and the antibody that is not bound by analyte in the sample will be captured by the analyte on the particles. Following incubation, the particles are separated magnetically and the enzyme activity in the supernatant is measured by the addition of o-nitrophenylgalactoside (ONPG). The enzyme activity is directly proportional to the analyte concentration in the original sample.

Here we report the immobilization of an antigen and an antibody on chromium dioxide magnetic particles and their application in digoxin and follitropin enzyme immunoassays.

II. MATERIALS AND METHODS

A. Materials

1. Instrumentation

We used manual pipettes: SMI Digital Adjust Micro/Pettor, Series A-K (Scientific Manufacturing Industries, Emeryville, CA 94608) or Titertek Digital Multichannel Pipet (Flow Laboratories, McLean, VA 22102), both of which typically exhibit SD of 0.2 μl at 20 μl.

Samples were incubated, mixed, and separated in one of two configurations: (a) Manual incubation in 12 × 75 mm polypropylene tubes in a waterbath (37 ± 0.1°C), manual mixing, and separation in a magnetic separation rack (Ciba-Corning Diagnostics, Medfield, MA 02052), followed by washing via aspiration at reduced pressure; (b) manual incubation in 8.8 × 4.5 mm polypropylene tubes in a waterbath (37 ± 0.5°C), manual mixing, and separation over a magnetic plate, followed by washing via aspiration with a multichannel manifold.

We used three modes of measurement: (a) spectrophotometric rate measurement of absorbance changes at 405 nm with a Cobas Bio® Automatic analyzer (Roche Diagnostic Systems, Nutley, NJ 07110). (b) turbidimetric measurement of chromium dioxide particle suspensions with a HP 8451A Diode Array Spectrophotometer (Hewlett Packard, Palo Alto, CA 94304) at 600 nm (1.0-cm-long cuvette); (c) fluorometric measurement of endpoint fluorescence in 96-well microtiter plates, with a MicroFLUOR™ reader (Dynatech Laboratories, Inc., Alexandria, VA 22314) at 365 nm (excitation) and 450 nm (emission): typical sensitivity, 10^{-8} mol of methylumbelliferone per liter; dynamic range, 0–4094 relative fluorescence units.

2. Reagents

We used the following substrate solutions: o-Nitrophenylgalactopyranoside (10 mmol/l) in HEPES buffer (0.25 mol/l, pH 7.7 at 25°C) containing 8.8 mmol/l of magnesium acetate and preservative; 4-methylumbelliferyl phosphate 1.0 mmol/l in diethanolamine buffer, 1 mol/l, pH 8.9 (25°C).

The wash buffer contained, per liter, 10 mmol of Tris (pH 7.0), 0.5 g of Tween 20 (polyoxyethylene). The quench reagent contained, per liter, 500 mmol of disodium EDTA, pH 8.9.

Digoxin antibody-β-galactosidase conjugate reagent was from Du Pont, part number 790772 (DuPont Company, Diagnostic Systems Division, Wilmington, DE 19898).

3. Samples and Standards

Digoxin calibrators (three levels) were obtained from Du Pont, part number 792022. The FSH calibrator was prepared by adding human follitropin (Radioassay Systems Laboratory, Inc., Carson, CA 90746) to horse serum and calibrated with reference to the World Health Organization's Second International Reference Preparation (2nd IRP-HMG).

For these studies we obtained fresh human serum samples and stored them frozen at $-20°C$ or $-70°C$.

B. Preparatory Procedures

1. Monoclonal Antibodies

BALB/c mice were immunized with follitropin or lutropin to obtain the alpha-specific or beta-specific clones. Spleen lymphocytes were fused with P3-NS1 1Ag4 mouse myeloma cells using polyethylene glycol by the protocol of Faze-kas de St. Groth and Scheidegger (6). The resulting clones were initially screened by ELISA, then by an RIA with iodinated FSH (Du Pont NEN Products). Clones were recloned and injected intraperitoneally into pristane-primed BALB/c mice. We purified the ascites on a protein A-Sepharose 4B column, eluting the bound antibodies with sodium citrate buffer (50 mmol/l, pH 3.0).

2. Alkaline Phosphatase-Conjugated Antibodies

Alkaline phosphatase (EC 3.13.1, from calf intestine, Boehringer Mannheim, Indianapolis, IN 46250) was activated with succinimidyl 4-(N-maleimidomethyl) cyclohexane-1-carboxylate (Pierce Chemical Co., Rockford, IL 61105) and coupled to sulfhydryl group-enriched IgG (4).

3. Chromium Dioxide Particles

Chromium dioxide particles were formed by a high-temperature, high-pressure oxidation-reduction reaction of chromic acid and chromic oxide (7). After stabilizing the particles by a reductive surface treatment (8) and coating them with a protective silica coating (9), we activated the particles by derivatizing the surface by silanization (10), incubating them with 50 g/l glutaraldehyde solution (11) for 3 h at room temperature, and washing them 10 times with phosphate buffer (10 mmol/l, pH 7.0).

4. Chromium Dioxide-Antibody Particles

Activated chromium dioxide particles, 50 g/l, were incubated overnight at room temperature with antibody 1 g/l in phosphate buffer (10 mmol/l, pH 7.0), containing 1 g bovine serum albumin per liter. We then washed the particles 10 times, diluted them to the proper assay concentration, and stored them in the same buffer at $4°C$.

5. Chromium Dioxide Particles Coated with Ouabain-
Bovine Serum Albumin (BSA)

Activated chromium dioxide particles, 25 g/l, were incubated overnight at room temperature with 1 g/l of ouabain-BSA in phosphate buffer (10 mmol/l, pH 7.0).

The ouabain-BSA was prepared according to the procedure of J. W. Freytag (5). After the incubation, we washed the particles 10 times with the phosphate buffer, containing 1.0 g of bovine serum albumin per liter. We then diluted the particles to the proper assay concentration and stored this in phosphate buffer (10 mmol/l, pH 7.0) containing 0.1% bovine serum albumin and 0.01% thimerosal as preservative.

C. Assay Procedures

1. FSH Assay

Add 50 μl sample, calibrator, or control to 50 μl of chromium dioxide-anti-FSH particles and 25 μl alkaline phosphatase-anti-βFSH conjugate; incubate for 20 min at 37°C. Then separate the reaction mixture components in the magnetic rack and remove the supernatant by aspiration. Wash the particles three times with 500 μl of the wash buffer. After the final wash, resuspend the particles and incubate in 200 μl substrate solution (4-methylumbelliferyl phosphate) for 4 min at 37°C, then add 300 μl of the quench reagent and mix. Again, separate the particles in the magnetic rack, and remove the supernatant and transfer it to a 96-well microtiter plate for fluorescence measurement in the microtiter plate reader. We converted the relative fluorescence to FSH concentration by using a linear function.

2. Digoxin Assay

Add 50 μl of water, 50 μl of sample, and 50 μl of digoxin antibody-β-galactosidase conjugate reagent in a test tube and incubate for 10 min at 37°C. To the mixture add 50 μl of ouabain-BSA coated chromium dioxide particles and incubate at 37°C for 5 min. The magnetic particles are separated in the magnetic rack and the supernatant is aspirated into a Cobas Bio® sample cup and assayed for enzyme activity on the Cobas-Bio using Rate Mode 2 at a wavelength of 405 nm. The enzyme concentration is directly proportional to the digoxin concentration in the samples.

III. RESULTS

A. Antigen Capture

A monoclonal antibody with high specificity and affinity for prostatic acid phosphatase was immobilized on both chromium dioxide particles and 6-mm diameter polystyrene beads. The amount of sample antigen captured from the solution phase onto the solid support (chromium dioxide particles or polystyrene bead) was measured as a function of capture-incubation time, using substrate (p-nitrophenyl phosphate) to measure the activity of the captured antigen.

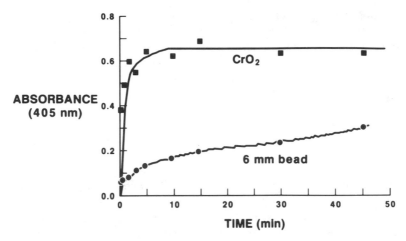

Figure 6 Antigen capture time course: chromium dioxide particles (■); 6-mm polystyrene bead (●).

As shown in Figure 6, greater than 90% of the sample antigen was captured in the first 3 min of the incubation period with chromium dioxide particles. A substantially smaller percentage ($< 20\%$) was captured by the polystyrene bead in 10 min. Furthermore, total capture by the bead was not achieved until > 20 h.

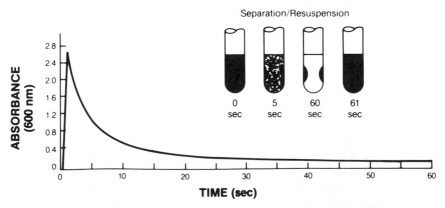

Figure 7 Magnetic separation and resuspension time course for chromium dioxide particles.

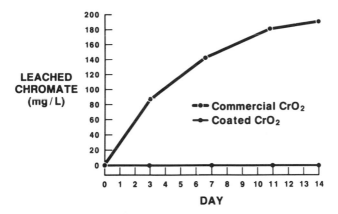

Figure 8   Relative stability of "magnetic tape" chromium dioxide particles (-•-) and stabilized "assay quality" chromium dioxide particles (-•-) at 37°C.

B. Separation/Resuspension Characteristics

The responsiveness of chromium dioxide particles to magnetic aggregation and resuspension was measured turbidimetrically. As shown in Figure 7, the particles exhibit excellent responsiveness to magnetic aggregation and resuspension, typically completing the entire process of separation and complete resuspension in less than 2 minutes.

C. Stability of Chromium Dioxide Particles

Hydrolytic stability, as measured by chromate leaching versus time, for magnetic tape particles and assay quality particles is shown in Figure 8. While the magnetic tape particles are highly unstable in solution, the specially coated assay

Table 1 FSH Assay Performance

	Reproducibility		
Mean (mIU/ml)	SD	% CV	N
8.5	0.78	9.2	20
26.4	0.73	2.8	20

Assay range: 0–200 mIU/ml
Recovery, $\bar{X}$, range: 104.4% (100.0–108.7%)

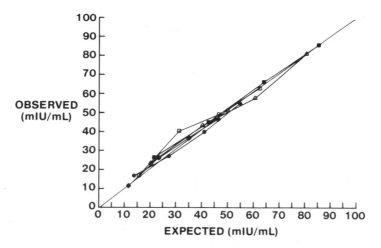

Figure 9 Parallelism of FSH assay: dilutions with zero calibrator (o), serum sample A (●), sample B (△), sample C (□), sample D (■), and sample E (♦).

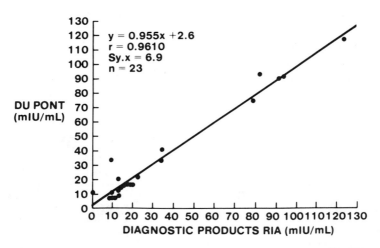

Figure 10 Correlation of FSH assay results by chromium dioxide particles and RIA.

Table 2 Digoxin Assay Performance

Mean (ng/ml)	Reproducibility		
	SD	% CV	N
0.62	0.02	2.7	20
1.20	0.02	1.8	20
2.53	0.06	2.4	20

Assay range: 0.2–5.0 ng/ml
Recovery, $\overline{X}$, Range: 100.6%, (97.8–103.8%)

quality particles are stable for > 14 days at 37°C and have demonstrated a shelf-life of over one year at 4°C.

D. FSH Assay

Standard curves exhibited an analytical range through 100 IU/l, standardized with the World Health Organization's Second International Reference Preparation. Analytical recovery was measured in three random sera by adding 10 IU/l

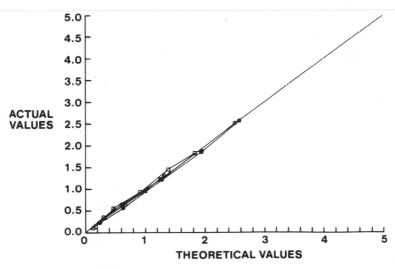

Figure 11 Parallelism of digoxin assay: dilution with zero calibrator (o), serum sample A (●), sample B (△), and sample C (□).

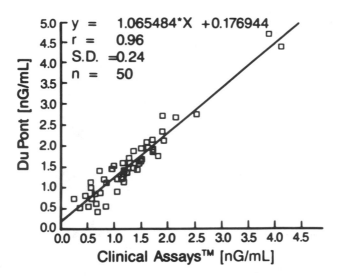

Figure 12 Correlation of digoxin assay results by chromium dioxide particles and RIA.

of FSH to each sample. The mean analytical recovery was 104.4% (range 100.0–108.7). Intra-assay precision (CV) for FSH in serum-based controls ranged from 2.8 to 9.2% at 26.4 and 8.8 IU/l, respectively (Table 1). Parallelism was determined by diluting each of five random sera (> 45 IU/l) with the zero calibrator. Each of the serum dilutions exhibit excellent parallelism with the standard curve (Fig. 9). The FSH assay correlated well (r=0.961) with the widely used RIA method, DPC double antibody FSH (Diagnostic Products Corporation, Los Angeles, CA 90045), and exhibited the following regression statistics: slope 0.955, intercept 2.6 IU/l, and standard error (Sy/x) 6.9 IU/l (Fig. 10).

E. Digoxin Assay

The assay range of the digoxin assay is 0.2 to 5.0 ng/ml, which is comparable to most assays. Recovery, an indication of method accuracy, was challenged by spiking ten random sera with digoxin. Recovery range was 98–104% with a mean of 101%. Intrarun precision was determined using commercial serum-based control products, showing 1.8 to 2.7% CV over the assay range, which is comparable to current state-of-the-art methods (Table 2). Parallelism of the digoxin method was demonstrated by diluting each of three random sera (> 3 ng/mL) with the zero calibrator. Each of the serum dilutions shows excellent parallelism with the standard curve (Fig. 11). Digoxin method correlation is excellent against the widely used Clinical Assays GammaCoat RIA method. The correlation coefficient is 0.96 with a slope of 1.07 for 50 patient samples covering the entire assay range (Fig. 12).

IV. DISCUSSION

The use of chromium dioxide particles as a solid support allowed us to develop very sensitive and rapid immunoassays. Chromium dioxide particles offer a significantly larger surface area than can be achieved with the more common solid supports, such as 6-mm diameter polystyrene beads, coated tubes, and microtiter plates. Each assay typically employs 50–250 μg of chromium dioxide particles. The higher surface area represented by this amount of chromium dioxide allows more immobilized antibody to be presented to the sample. Because the capture mechanism is a bimolecular reaction, the law-of-mass-action dictates that the kinetics must occur faster when the concentration of one or both of the reactants is increased. The capture kinetics are further enhanced, with immobilized species, when the solid phase can be intimately mixed throughout the solution, thus reducing the mean path of diffusion of the individual reactants. The final result is a faster turnaround of test results: < 30 min for FSH and < 15 min for measuring digoxin.

The special coating applied to magnetic tape chromium dioxide particles serves several purposes in the production of assay quality particles. First, it prevents chromate leaching and improves hydrolytic stability. Second, it reduces the magnetic aggregation of the particles when exposed to a magnetic field. Third, it produces a surface that can be easily modified to reduce nonspecific binding. Finally, it provides a functional surface for the covalent coupling of antigens and antibodies, which improves the stability of the assays and yields a high protein uptake capacity.

The magnetic responsiveness of chromium dioxide particles offer optimal utility in solid-phase immunoassays. Although they are ferromagnetic, the particles exhibit low remanent magnetism, thus allowing repeated separation and resuspension for incubation, washing, and measurement steps. The ability to optimally wash the particles, along with the ability to easily modify the surface, is responsible for low nonspecific binding and minimal matrix effects. These characteristics are responsible for the excellent parallelism and recovery exhibited by each of the assays.

The coated particles also provide a special feature which allows us to treat the particle slurry as a liquid reagent for precise delivery. Although all of the assays in this paper require delivery of slurries by manual or semiautomated pipetting devices, the assay results demonstrate excellent precision. In addition, the particle support has been used with both spectrophotometric and fluorometric detection systems. These results demonstrate that the technology is highly flexible and applicable to a variety of assay formats, from manual to fully automated.

In summary, we have demonstrated a wide range of applications for the chromium dioxide particle technology. The performance of FSH and digoxin assays have been shown in detail. Assays using the same technology for many other analytes such as hormones, cancer markers, and infectious disease markers have also been published elsewhere (4). Good precision and accuracy, exemplified by excellent recovery, parallelism, and correlation, were demonstrated with assay times that represent a fraction of the time required by other isotopic or nonisotopic methods for these analytes.

REFERENCES

1. Al-Djuaili, E. A. S., Forrest, G. C., Edwards, C. R. W., and Landon, J. (1979). Evaluation and application of magnetizable charcoal for separation in radioimmunoassays. *Clin. Chem. 25*:1402–1405.
2. Nargessi, R. D., Ackland, J., Hassan, M., Forrest, G. C., Smith, D. S., and Landon, J. (1979). Magnetizable solid-phase fluoroimmunoassay of thyroxine by a sequential addition technique. *Clin. Chem. 26*:1701–1703.
3. Lau, H. P., Yang, E. K., and Jacobson, H. W. (1987). Surface composition of chromium dioxide particles for use in magnetic affinity supports in diagnostic assays. U.S. Patent 4,661,408.
4. Birkmeyer, R. C., Diaco, R., Hutson, D. K., Lau, H. P., Miller, W. K., Neelkantan, N. V., Pankratz, T. J., Tseng, S. Y., Vickery, D. K., and Yang, E. K. (1987). Application of novel chromium dioxide magnetic particles to immunoassay development. *Clin. Chem. 33*:1543–1547.
5. Freytag, J. W., Lau, H. P., and Wadsley, J. J. (1984). Affinity-column-mediated immunoenzymometric assays: Influence of affinity-column ligand and valence of antibody-enzyme conjugates. *Clin. Chem. 30*:1494–1498.
6. Fazekas de St. Groth, S., and Scheidegger, D. (1980). Production of monoclonal antibodies: strategy and tactics. *J. Immunol. Methods 35*:1–21.
7. Ingraham, J. N., and Swoboda, T. J. (1960). Antimony-modified chromium dioxide, ferromagnetic compositions and their use. U.S. Patent 2,923,683.
8. Bottjer, W. G. (1970). Ingersoll HG. Stabilized ferromagnetic chromium dioxide. U.S. Patent 3,512,930.
9. Iler, R. K. (1959). Product comprising a skin of dense, amorphous silica bound upon a core of another solid material and process of making same. U.S. Patent 2,885,366.
10. Weetall, H. H. (1976). Covalent coupling methods for inorganic supports. *Methods Enzymol. 44*:134–148.
11. Klibanov, A. M. (1983). Immobilized enzymes and cells as practical catalysts. *Science 219*:722–727.

11

Use of Coated Latex Particles for Identifcation and Localization of *Candida albicans* Cell Surface Receptors and for Detection of Related Circulating Antigens and/or Antibodies in Patient Sera and Urine

RAYMOND ROBERT, GUY TRONCHIN, VERONIQUE ANNAIX, ABDELHAMID BOUALI, and JEAN-MARCEL SENET
UFR des Sciences Médicales et Pharmaceutiques-Section Pharmacie, Laboratoire d'Immunologie-Parasitologie-Mycologie, Angers, France

I. INTRODUCTION

Fungal adherence has become one of the most active areas of study in the field of mycological ecology. Among the 81 known species of candida, only one tenth can be pathogenic for humans, *Candida albicans* itself being responsible for most of the pathologic processes. A saprophyte common to the gastrointestinal tract and mucosal surfaces, *Candida albicans* manifests at these levels as blastospores which multiply by budding. When involved in a pathogenic host tissue colonization, mycelial phases appear simultaneously with the blastospore forms. This process of infection can be envisioned as a stepwise process in which the fungus must first adhere to a tissue surface (1-10). This phenomenon involves most certainly cell to cell interactions in which precise host cell surface components correspond and react specifically with a surface receptor of the parasite. This interaction must be strong enough to allow the fixation of the fungus on the tissue surface, preventing its elimination by the biological fluids which constantly bathe tissue surface. Although much research has been conducted in this area, little information is available on the exact identity of the linking molecules at the surface level of the yeast. Conversely, many host components such as complement (11), fibronectin (12), and fibrinogen (13–17) have been suggested as the host-binding site for the fungus.

In our laboratory, we have demonstrated that *Candida albicans* possesses a 68 kD mannoprotein receptor which is able to bind itself firmly to fibrinogen (6,13,14,17).

The study and identification of surface receptors are usually made with molecules labeled with fluorochrome enzymes, colloidal gold, ferritin, and substances, depending on the technique used.

This chapter describes our own findings using particulate markers previously coated with the protein to be studied for its linking ability. This study has been conducted with protein-coated latex particles (CLP) in order to identify and localize receptors for these proteins on the upper layer of *Candida albicans* by means of electron and photonic microscopy. Concanavalin A-CLP were used for identification of mannan receptors. Fibrinogen-CLP or a two-layer reactive (anti-fibrinogen-protein A-CLP) permits the localization of a fibrinogen receptor.

Furthermore, the agglutination ability of CLP by either antigens or antibodies is very convenient for diagnostic purposes.

II. MATERIALS AND METHODS

A. Organisms and Culture Conditions

Candida albicans strain 1066 (serotype A) originally isolated from a case of *Candida septicemia* was used throughout. Cultures were maintained by subculture on Sabouraud dextrose agar (Merck) twice a month. Organisms were grown either as blastospores on this medium at 37°C for 24 h or as germ tube and mycelium on 199 medium at 37°C for 2 and 24 h or 72 h, respectively. They were then harvested by centrifugation and washed in phosphate-buffered saline (PBS) at pH 7.2.

B. Extract Preparation

Culture supernatants (CS) were prepared by centrifugation (40,000 g for 30 min) from 48 h culture at 37°C in medium 199. Mannan was extracted from whole blastospore by the method of Peat et al. (18). *Candida albicans* fibrinogen receptor (CFR) was isolated from the culture media by means of affinity chromatography using fibrinogen-coated ultragel column as previously described (6).

C. Preparation and Purification of Antisera

Rabbits injected subcutaneously with 10^6 blastospores, killed with 0.2% formaldehyde, at 10-day intervals, were bled 10 days after the fourth injection. The IgG was isolated by DEAE trisacryl chromatography.

Antimannan antibodies from the IgG fraction were purified by chromatography on mannan Sepharose [purified mannan was coupled to epoxy-activated Sepharose 6 B Beads according to the procedure indicated by the manufacturer (Pharmacia Fine Chemicals)]. IgG fraction to rabbit anti-CFR was depleted of most of its antimannan antibodies by chromatography on mannan–Sepharose.

D. Reagents

Blue latex particles (LP) were kindly provided as a 10% suspension by Rhône-Poulenc (Aubervilliers, France). Three kinds of LP were used: (1) carboxylated polystyrene LP 0.3 μm diameter, (2) carboxylated polystyrene LP 0.8 μm diameter, (3) hydroxylated polystyrene LP 0.8 μm diameter.

The following materials were purchased from commerical sources: Concanavalin A, epoxy-activated Sepharose 6B (Pharmacia Fine Chemicals, Sweden) Protein A, DEAE-trisacryl, activated ultrogel, (IBF, Villeneuve la Garenne, France). Rabbit anti-human fibrinogen, Fibrinogen free of factor XIII (Diagnostica, Stago, France). Fluorescein isothiocyanate conjugated goat anti-rabbit IgG (Cappel, Cooper Biomedical). 1-Ethyl-3.3-dimethyl amino propyl carbodiimide HCl (EDC) (Merck, France). Colloidal gold (Janssen Pharmaceutica, Sweden). P-1.4-Benzoquinone (Fluka, AG, Sweden).

Human fibrinogen was found to contain a small amount of fibronectin and then was further purified by successive passage through ultrogel columns substituted with gelatin and heparin (IBF, France).

E. Preparation of LP Conjugates

1. Coupling of Proteins to Carboxylated LP

To 100 μl of 10% latex suspension in 0.14M NaCl containing 0.01M borate HCl pH 8.5 (BBS) were added 1 ml of protein in BBS (fibrinogen 0.5 mg/ml, Concanavalin A 0.25 mg/ml, protein A 0.25 mg/ml, CFR 0.2 mg/ml, antimannan antibodies 0.1 mg/ml) and 0.5 mg of EDC (19,20). The mixture was incubated for 2 h at 37°C. After three washings with 4 ml of BBS containing 1% bovine serum albumin (BBS-BSA), the LP were resuspended in 10 ml of BBS-BSA containing 0.1% Tween 20 for cell surface labeling in light and scanning electron microscopy) or in 1 ml of PBS–BSA (for macroscopic agglutination).

2. Coupling of Mannan to Hydroxylated LP (21–23)

To 35 mg of mannan in 8 ml of 0.1M phosphate buffer at pH 7 were added 2 ml of ethanol containing 60 mg of p-benzoquinone. The mixture was kept in darkness for 1 h at room temperature. The activated mannan was then mixed with 45 ml of methanol. The precipitate was collected by centrifugation (900 x g for 15 min), washed with methanol and acetone, and then dried in a vacuum desiccator. To 0.5 ml of hydroxylated LP at 10% was added 0.1 ml of activated mannan

(10 mg/ml in NaHCO$_3$ 0.1M). The suspension was incubated 1 h at 37°C. The LP was washed with PBS and suspended in 5 ml of PBS–BSA.

F. Scanning Electron Microscopy (SEM)

Direct technique: 0.5 ml of cells (10^7/ml) was incubated with 0.5 ml of proteins conjugated with LP. The cells were harvested after 30 min of incubation and washed three times with PBS containing 0.1% Tween 20.

Sandwich technique: (1) cells (0.5 ml) were treated with 0.5 ml of fibrinogen at 0.4 mg/ml in PBS. Cells were then washed in PBS and treated with 0.5 ml of rabbit anti-human fibrinogen at 1/100 dilution in PBS for 30 min. After several washings, protein A-LP was added to the cells for 30 min. (2) Cells (0.5 ml) were treated with 0.5 ml of antimannan antibodies for 30 min at room temperature. After washing, cells were incubated with protein A-LP (30 min at room temperature). The organisms were fixed with 2.5% glutaraldehyde at pH 7.4 in sodium cacodylate buffer 0.1M. Following washings in distilled water and dehydration, cells were dried at the critical point, metal-coated with gold-palladium, and examined with a JSM 35 C jeol microscope. In some experiments cells were observed under a Nikon microscope equipped for differential interference.

G. Macroscopic Agglutination on Glass Plates

For detection of antibodies to mannan and CFR, mannan latex and CFR latex were suspended at 10% in PBS–BSA. On the glass plate were placed 20 μl of serum dilution (1/10 with PBS BSA) and 20 μl of latex. The drops were mixed and the plate gently rotated by hand for 5 min until blue-colored masses were obtained with positive serum.

For detection of mannan antigen, latex particles coated with antimannan antibodies were used at 10% in PBS–BSA, and sera or urine were diluted (1/3) with phosphate buffer 0.15M pH 8.6.

In human studies, the sera and urine were collected from 30 blood donors and 16 patients with systemic candidiasis. In animal studies, 5 rabbits were inoculated intravenously with (10^7 to 10^9) blastospores suspended in 1 ml NaCl 0.15M. Sera and urine were collected daily until death 2 days after injection.

H. Overlay Procedure

Immunofluorescence testing had been performed with a double-sandwich procedure (fibrinogen-rabbit antifibrinogen antibodies-fluorescein isothiocyanate conjugate goat anti-rabbit IgG (14). Scanning electron microscopy using fibrinogen gold complexes were performed as described previously (17,24).

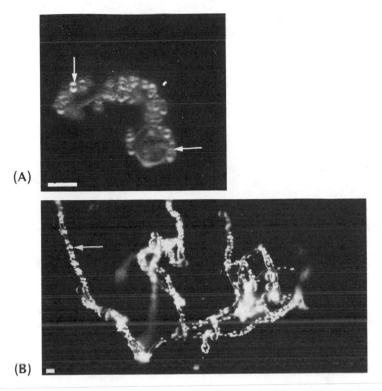

Figure 1 Localization of mannan on the surface of *Candida albicans* by direct method as observed by light microscopy. Concanavalin-CLP were dispersed on germ tube (A – top arrow), blastospore (A – bottom arrow), and pseudohyphae (B – arrow). Bar = 5 μm.

III. RESULTS

A. Mannan Cell Surface Labeling

Light microscopic observations evince that Concanavalin–CLP (0.8 μm diameter) incubated with *Candida albicans* fix every stage of the fungus: blastospores, germ tubes pseudohyphae, and mycelium (Fig. 1). This fixation is inhibited in the presence of α-D-glucopyranoside (0.1M). Similar results are obtained with antimannan–CLP (Fig. 2).

B. Candida Fibrinogen Receptor Localization

Fibrinogen–CLP (0.3 μm and 0.8 μm diameter) bind closely to the germ tube surface and 24-h old *Candida albicans* mycelium. On the contrary, there is no fixation on the blastospore (Fig. 3). Electron microscopy confirms the photonic

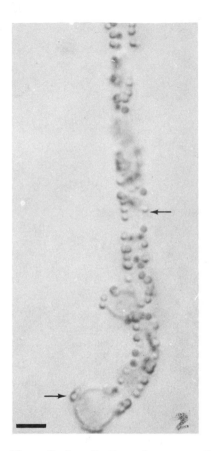

Figure 2 Localization of mannan with antimannan CLP. Blastospore (left arrow) and mycelium (right arrow) were labeled. Bar = 5 μm.

observations and shows in sharper detail the relation between the *Candida albicans* and the CLP. Fibrinogen–CLP adhere as clusters to the *Candida* cell very strongly. Within a single pseudomycelium there are areas that bind CLP and those that do not (Fig. 4).

Fibrinogen–CLP (0.8 μm diameter) adherence to the tip of pseudohyphae is very obvious, the *Candida* cell body (Fig. 5), is almost completely covered by clusters of CLP.

At 72 h, mycelium (Fig. 6) surface labeling was heterogeneous and weak compared to newly formed germ tubes or 24-h old pseudohyphae. On older mycelium none or few CLP can be seen.

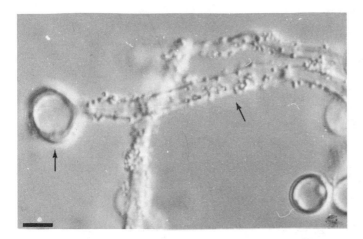

Figure 3 Surface labeling by fibrinogen CLP (0.3 μm diameter) as observed by light microscopy. Label appeared on mycelium (right arrow). The left arrow indicate the absence of LP on the blastospore. Bar = 5μm.

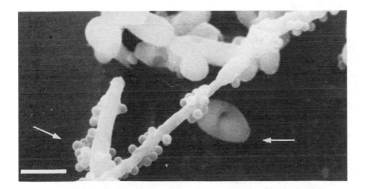

Figure 4 Localization of fibrinogen receptor on the surface of *Candida albicans* by fibrinogen–CLP as detected by scanning electron microscopy. The cell surface of mycelium (left arrow) was labeled whereas blastospores (right arrow) were free of marking. Bar = 5 μm.

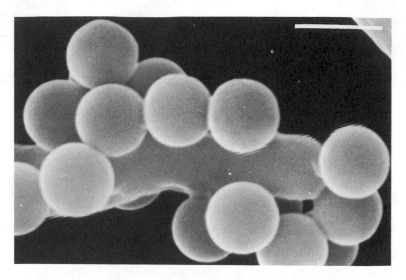

Figure 5   Scanning electron microscopy of germ tube labeled with fibrinogen-CLP. Bar = 1 μm.

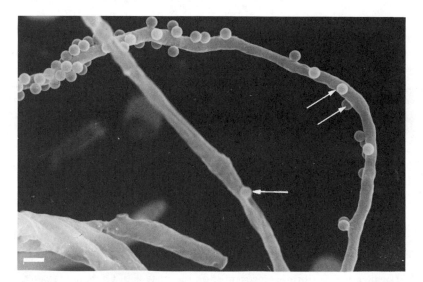

Figure 6   Binding of fibrinogen–CLP to 72-h old mycelium. Note the weakness or the absence of labeling on older mycelium (arrows). Bar = 1 μm.

Table 1 Detection of Antibodies to *Candida albicans* (Mannan and CFR) by Macroscopic Agglutination in Sera of Blood Donors and Patients with Systemic Candidiasis

	Blood donors		Patients with systemic candidiasis	
Macroscopic agglutination	+	−	+	−
Antibodies to mannan	28	2	15	1
Antibodies to CFR	25	5	16	0

A double-sandwich technique (antifibrinogen-protein A–CLP) demonstrated the fixation of soluble fibrinogen on the surface of germ tube and mycelial phases of *Candida albicans* but, as previously observed in the case of fibrinogen-CLP, there is no fixation upon the surface of blastospores (data not shown).

C. Antimannan and Anti-CFR Antibody Detection

Agglutination tests made with mannan and CFR–CLP revealed that most of the patients tested, whether healthy controls (blood donors) or patients suffering from any visceral candidiasis, show positive tests (Table 1).

D. Mannan Antigen Detection in Serum and Urine

Using a reverse agglutination technique with antimannan antibody–CLP, no mannan can be found in the serum and urine of healthy people, whereas mannan antigen has been detected in the serum of two patients and in the urine of 10 of 16 patients with a systemic candidiasis infection (Table 2).

Table 2 Detection of Mannan Antigen in Sera and Urine of Blood Donors and Patients Infected by *Candida albicans*

	Blood donors		Patients with systemic candidiasis	
Macroscopic agglutination	+	−	+	−
Mannan in serum	0	30	2	14
Mannan in urine	0	30	10	6

Table 3 Detection of Mannan Antigen in Sera-Infected Rabbit by Macroscopic Agglutination

	Time after *Candida albicans* infection							
Rabbit	Day 0	Day 2	Day 3	Day 4	Day 5	Day 8	Day 10	Day 12
1	−	+	Dead					
2	−	−	Dead					
3	−	−	+	+	+	Dead		
4	−	−	−	−	−	Dead		
5	−	−	+	+	+	+	+	Dead

Detection of mannan antigenemia in rabbits experimentally infected with candida is not very sensitive to agglutination testing; only 3 of 5 tested rabbits showed positive (Table 3). On the other hand, mannan could be detected from the second day in the urine of all rabbits tested (Table 4).

IV. DISCUSSION

Although CLP have been used for diverse purposes (25–27), medical mycology has not yet widely benefited from this technique.

This chapter focused mainly on the study of surface components of *Candida albicans*. We have demonstrated that the use of CLP can compete with more conventional methods. Light microscopic observations show that fibrinogen-CLP, when incubated with different stages of *Candida albicans*, bind specifically

Table 4 Result of Macroscopic Agglutination for Detection of Mannan Antigen in Rabbit Urine

	Time after *Candida albicans* infection						
Rabbit	Day 0	Day 2	Day 4	Day 6	Day 8	Day 10	Day 12
1	−	+	Dead				
2	−	+	Dead				
3	−	+	ND	+	Dead		
4	−	+	+	ND	Dead		
5	−	+	+	+	ND	+	Dead

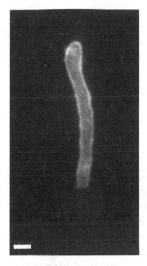

(A)

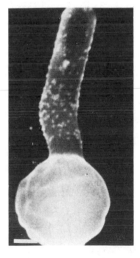

(B)

Figure 7 Immunofluorescence of germ tube of *Candida albicans* stained with fibrinogen (A). Scanning electron microscopy using fibrinogen gold complex. Gold particles were unequally dispersed on the germ tube surface (B). Bar = 1 µm.

to the germ tube forms making the localization of a fibrinogen receptor possible at this level, whereas no fixation can be seen on the surface of the mother blastospores (Fig. 3). The utilization of a double-sandwich procedure (antifibrinogen-protein A-CLP) is well adapted to the study of the linking of soluble fibrinogen molecules to the yeast surface and confirms the results obtained with fibrinogen-CLP. Similar results are obtained with more complicated and time-consuming immunofluorescence technique (Fig. 7a). CLP can be conveniently used for scanning electron microscopic observations (Figs. 4–6). When compared to scanning electron microscopy using fibrinogen coupled with gold particles (Fig. 7b), fibrinogen-CLP procedure shows very similar results which are more easily discernible.

When applied to diagnostic purposes, rapid agglutination tests with CLP have the advantage of being manageable either for antibodies or antigens detection. In our study, antimannan antibodies-CLP allow the detection of mannan antigen in urine as has been already demonstrated for patients with systemic candidiasis and for experimentally infected rabbits. However, mannan antigenemia often escapes detection (28–30). In the case of antibody detection, slide agglutination of mannan or CFR-CLP gives very similar results to those obtained with other serological technique (21,22,31). Most people, whether they are healthy or affected by candidiasis have a more or less stable concentration of antimannan antibodies in their serum. This is due to the ubiquitous status of the fungus.

To conclude, it might be said that coupling covalently various molecules to LP, thus conferring to the latter a new identity is of capital interest. It has proved very convenient to many purposes in the field of biological investigations. This technique covers a wide field of applications ranging from such fundamental approaches as the study of molecular mechanisms of adherence to diagnostic methods such as rapid testing or even taxonomic studies.

When taking into account its encouraging performances, this method is destined to be used with increasing profit in the future.

REFERENCES

1. Douglas, L. J., Houston, J. G., and McCourtie, J. (1981). Adherence of *Candida albicans* to human buccal epithelial cells after growth on different carbon sources. *FEMS Microbiol. Letter 12*:241–243.
2. Douglas, L. J., and McCourtie, J. (1981). Adherence of *Candida albicans* to denture acrylic as affected by changes in cell-surface composition. In *Current Developments in Yeast Research*, Pergamon Press, Toronto, 375–380.
3. Kimura, L. H., and Pearsall, N. N. (1980). Relationship between germination of *Candida albicans* and increased adherence to human buccal epithelial cells. *Infect. Immun. 28*:464–468.
4. King, R. D., Lee, J. C., and Morris, A. L. (1980). Adherence of *Candida albicans* and other *Candida* species to mucosal epithelial cells. *Infect. Immun. 27*:667–674.

5. Klotz, S. A., Drutz, D. J., Harrison, J. L., and Huppert, M. (1983). Adherence and penetration of vascular endothelium by *Candida* yeasts. *Infect. Immun.* *42*:374–384.

6. Robert, R., Senet, J. M., Tronchin, G., and Bouali, A. (1988). *Candida* antigens and their role in adherence mechanisms. *First Internatinal Symposium on Fungal Antigens*. Inst. Pasteur de Paris, Plenum, New York.

7. Rotrosen, D., Edwards, J. E., Moore, J., Adler, J., Cohen, A. M., and Green, I. (1983). Pathogenesis of hematogenous candidiasis: adherence of *Candida* species to vascular endothelium and mechanisms of endothelial cell invasion. *Clin. Res. 31*:374A.

8. Rotrosen, D., Edwards, J. E., Gibson, T. R., Moore, J., Cohen, A. M., and Green, I. (1985). Adherence of *Candida* to cultured vascular endothelial cells: mechanisms of attachment and endothelial cell penetration. *J. Infect. Dis. 152*:1264–1274.

9. Segal, E., Sorola, A., and Schechter, A. (1984). Correlative relationship between adherence of *Candida albicans* to human vaginal epithelial cells in vitro and *Candida vaginitis*. *Sabouraudia 22*:191–200.

10. Sobel, J. D., Muller, G., Myers, P. G., Kaye, D., and Levison, M. E. (1981). Adherence of *Candida albicans* to human vaginal and buccal epithelial cells. *J. Infect. Dis. 143*:76–82.

11. Edwards, J. E., Jr., Gaither, T. A., O'Shea, J. J., Rotrosen, D., Lawley, T. J., Wright, S. A., Frank, M. M., and Green, I. (1986). Expression of specific binding sites on *Candida* with functional and antigenic characteristics of human complement receptors. *J. Immunol. 137*(11).3577 3583

12. Skerl, K. G., Calderone, R. A., Segal, E., and Sreevalsan, T. (1983). In vitro binding of *Candida albicans* yeast cells to human fibronectin. *Can. J. Microbiol. 30*:221–227.

13. Bouali, A., Robert, R., Tronchin, G., and Senet, J. M. (1986). Binding of human fibrinogen to *Candida albicans* in vitro: a preliminary study. *Sabouraudia 24*:345–348.

14. Bouali, A., Robert, R., Tronchin, G., and Senet, J. M. (1987). Characterization of binding of human fibrinogen to the surface of germ-tube and mycelium of *Candida albicans*. *J. Gen. Microbiol. 133*:545–551.

15. Maisch, P. A., and Calderone, R. A. (1980). Adherence of *Candida albicans* to a fibrin-platelet-matrix formed in vitro. *Infect. Immun. 27*:650–656.

16. Maisch, P. A., and Calderone, R. A. (1981). Role of surface mannan in the adherence of *Candida albicans* to fibrin-platelet clots formed in vitro. *Infect. Immun. 32*:92–97.

17. Tronchin, G., Robert, R., Bouali, A., and Senet, J. M. (1987). Immunocytochemical localization of in vitro binding of human fibrinogen to *Candida albicans* germ tube and mycelium. *Ann. Inst. Pasteur/Microbiol. 138*: 177–187.

18. Peats, S., Whelan, W. J., and Edwards, T. E. (1961). Polysaccharides of baker's yeast. I.V. mannan. *J. Chem. Soc. 1*:29.

19. Quash, G., Roch, A. M., Niveleau, A., Grange, J., Keolouangkhot, T., and
    Huppert, J. (1978). The preparation of latex particles with covalently
    bound polyamines, IgG and measles agglutinines and their use in visual ag-
    glutination tests. *J. Immunol. Methods 22*:165–174.
20. Rembraum, A., Margel, S., and Levy, J. (1978). Polyglutaraldehyde: A new
    reagent for coupling proteins to microspheres and for labeling cell surface
    receptors. *J. Immunol. Methods 24*:239–250.
21. Robert, R., Siraudeau, J. J., and Senet, J. M. (1978). Diagnostic des can-
    didoses: recherche d'anticorps antimannane et d'antigène mannane circulant
    par hemaglutination indirecte (HAI) et inhibition de l'hemagglutination
    indirecte (INH BAI). *Bull. Soc. Myc. Méd. Tome VIII 2*:205–208.
22. Robert, R., Leynia de la Jarrige, P., Builbert, F., Chabasse, D., Senet, J. M.,
    and Hocquet, P. (1978). Valeur de la recherche d'anticorps antimannanes
    par hemagglutination indirecte dans le diagnostic des candidoses. *Bull. Soc.
    Bull. Soc. Myc. Méd. Tome VIII 2*:205–208.
23. Ternynck, T., and Avrameas, S. (1976). A new method using P. benzo-
    quinone for coupling antigens and anti-bodies to marker substances. *Ann.
    Immunol. (I.P.) 127*:197–208.
24. Horisberger, M. (1981). Colloidal gold: A cytochemical marker for light and
    fluorescent microscopy and for transmission and scanning electron micro-
    scopy. *Gold. Bull. 14*:90–94.
25. Gonda, M. A., Gilgen, M. A., Oroszlan, S., Hager, H., and Hsu, K. C. (1978).
    Immunolatex spheres for cell and virion surface labeling in the electron
    microscope. *Virology 86*:572–576.
26. Margel, S., Beitler, U., and Ofarim, M. (1982). Polyacrolein microspheres
    as a new tool in cell biology. *J. Cell. Sci. 56*:157–175.
27. Molday, R. S., and Maher, P. (1980). A review of cell surface markers and
    labeling techniques for scanning electron microscopy. *J. Histochem. 12*:
    273–315.
28. Robert, R., Leynia de la Jarrige, P., Guilbert, F., Chabasse, D., Senet, J.
    M., and Hocquet, P. (1979). Diagnostic des candidoses: recherche d'AG
    mannanes et d'immuncomplexes (AG Mannane-AC antimannane) dans le
    sang et les urines. *Bull. Soc. Myc. Méd. Tome VIII 2*:209–214.
29. Warren, R. C., Bartlett, A., Bidwell, D. E., Richardson, M. D., Voller, A.,
    and White, L. O. (1977). Diagnosis of invasive candidosis by enzyme im-
    munoassay of serum antigen. *Br. Med. J. 1*:1183–1185.
30. Weiner, M. H., and Yount, W. (1976). Mannan antigenemia in the diagnosis
    of invasive candida infections. *J. Chim. Invest. 58*:1045–1053.
31. Edge, G., and Pepys, J. (1976). Rasts Test avec des antigenes proteiniques
    et polysaccharidiques et des cellules lavees. *Rev. France. allergol. 16*:251–255.

Index

A

Adriamycin (AD), 76-80, 82
  chemical structure, 76
  drug-antibody conjugation, 76-80
Alkylating agents
  chlorambucil (CBL), 82-84, 88
  N-acetyl-melphalan, 82-85
Anthracycline, 77-80
  idarubicin, derivative of, 79-80,
    82, 87, 88
Amino acids, 43-44
Antibodies (*see also* Monoclonal
    antibodies):
  anti-idiotypic, 17, 20-23
  antimanna antibody-CLP, 225, 228
  antitumor activity, 9-11
  chimeric, 11-13
  chromium dioxide, 201-215
  conjugation to drugs, 76-83
  covalent coupling, 123-124, 155-

[Antibodies]
  184, 188-198, 203
  enzyme conjugate, 188-198
  immunoreactivity, 103-106, 109
  oligosaccharide linked, 101, 109
  reactivity, 57
  titers, 171, 174-179, 182-183
Antibody conjugates (*see* Immuno-
    conjugates, Immunotoxins, and
    Radiolabeled MAb)
Antibody-dependent cellular cyto-
    toxicity (ADCC), 9-13
Anti-CD5 T101, 44, 46-48
Anti-CFR, 225
Anti-CMV, 171, 174-175
Antigens:
  CD5, 48
  chromium dioxide, 201-215
  covalent coupling, 123-124, 155-
    184, 188-198, 203

[Antigens]
  gp 72, 56, 58, 64-65
  gp 95, 4
  idiotype-specific, 7-8
  mannan antigen, 225-226, 228
  melanoma-associated, 3
  p97, 3-7, 18-21
  p175, 21-22
  shared, 8
  Thy 1.2, 50
Anti-idiotypic (see under Antibody)
Anti-p97, 3-7, 18
Anti-PIV, 176-179
Anti-Thy 1.2, 45, 50-51

B

B72.3, 103-104, 106-107, 113-116
B-galactosidase, 188-198, 206-207
  polymerization of, 188-198
212Bi (see Bismuth-212)
Biodistribution, 68, 88, 107-109
Bismuth-212, 110-116
B-lymphoma (see Leukemia cell
  lines)
Bone marrow, transplantation, 48,
  137-147
Bone marrow purging, 137-147
  chemical methods, 138-141
  immunological methods, 139-141,
  145-147
  physical separation, 138
Bovine serum albumin (BSA), 156,
  188, 208-209
BSA (see Bovine serum albumin)

C

C3b, 120-133
Candida albicans cell surface receptors, 217-228
  binding with CLP, 221-226, 228
  fibrinogen receptor (CFR), 218-
  228
  localization of CFR, 221-223, 228

CD5, 48
Cell line LS174T (see LS174T cell
  line)
Chelators:
  diethylenetriaminepentaacetic
  acid (DTPA), 101-107, 110-116
  with Bismuth-212, 110-116
  with Indium-111, 56, 103-104,
  110-111, 114-115
Chlorambucil (CBL), 82-84, 88
  chemical structure, 82
  drug-antibody conjugation, 82-84,
  88
Chromium dioxide, 201-215
  hydrolytic stability, 203, 211, 213
CMV (see Cytomegalovirus)
Cobra venom factor (CVF), 120, 132
Colon carcinomas 56, 79-80, 114-
  116
Colorectal carcinomas, 54-56, 61-62
Complement:
  C3, 120
  C3b, 120-133
  crosslinking, 121-124, 128, 129
  cytotoxocity and binding, 121
  mediated killing, 128-131
Complement-dependent cytotoxicity
  (CDC), 9-13, 121
Complement-dependent lysis, 128-
  131, 139-141, 145-147
Conjugation to antibody:
  of adriamycin, 76-80
  of B-galactosidase, 188-198, 206-
  207
  of chlorambucil, 82-84, 88
  of daunomycin, 56, 67
  of GYK-DTPA, 101-107
  of HRP, 190-191
  of idarubicin, 79-80, 87, 88
  of methotrexate, 57-59, 61, 67-69
  of N-acetyl-melphalan, 82-84
  of ricin A chain, 41-46, 62-69
Covalent coupling, 123-124, 155-
  184, 203 (see also Site-specific
  coupling)

Covalently linked polymerized enzyme-antibody conjugate, 188-198
Cytomegalovirus (CMV), 170-175, 178-179, 182-183

D

Daunomycin, 16, 56, 67
DDIA (see Double-determinant immunoassay)
Delayed-type hypersensitivity (DTH), 16, 18-22
Diethylenetriaminepentaacetic acid (DTPA), 101-107, 110-116
Digoxin enzyme immunoassay, 206-207, 209, 213-215
Double-determinant immunoassay (DDIA), 4-5
DTPA (see Diethylenetriaminepentaacetic acid)

E

EIA (see Radioimmunoassay)
ELISA type assay, 103, 170-175, 178-179, 181-184
  OCA ELISA, 171, 174, 178-179, 181, 183
Enzyme immunometric assay (EIA) (see Radioimmunoassay)

F

Fab, 46-48, 162
Fab', 188-189, 190-198
  B-galactosidase conjugate, 189, 191-198
  horseradish peroxidase (HRP) conjugate, 190-198
Fab fragment, 5-6, 14
F(ab)'2, 46-47, 92-93, 189
Factor B, 119, 129
Factor I, 119-120
Factor H, 119-120, 130, 132

Follicle-stimulating hormone (FSH) enzyme immunoassay, 206-214 48.7, 6
FSH (see Follicle-stimulating hormone)

G

Glutaraldehyde, 121-123, 157-158, 188, 201, 204, 206, 208
  crosslinking with, 121-123
  hydrazone formation, 162
  peptide bond formation, 163
  agglutination tests, 165
Glycoproteins, 3, 21, 66, 120, 161-184
gp 72, 56, 58, 64-65
gp 95, 4
GYK-DTPA (see Diethylenetriaminepentaacetic acid)

H

2H7, 12 13
Haptens, 165, 177, 181, 182
Heterobifunctional reagents (see N-succinimidyl-3-(2-pyridyidithio)
Horseradish peroxidase (HRP), 188, 190-191, 197-198
  polymerization of, 190-191, 198
HRP (see Horseradish peroxidase)
HSA (see Human serum albumin)
HSA-monensin, 46-47, 50-51
Human cell lines (see Target cell lines)
Human serum albumin (HSA), 56-62, 67-69, 103, 196-197 (see also 791T/36)

I

125I (see Iodine-125)
131I (see Iodine-131)
Idarubicin, 79-80, 82, 87, 88-89
  chemical structure 79

[Idarubicin]
  drug-antibody conjugation, 79-80,
    87, 88
IEF (see Isoelectric focusing)
Imaging, 5-6, 107-109
IL-2, 3, 10, 16
Immunoassay (see Radioimmuno-
    assay)
Immunocomplexes, 175-181
  PVI, 176-177, 179, 183
Immunoconjugates (see also Immu-
    notoxins and specific drugs)
  adriamycin, 76-80, 82
  B-galactosidase, 188-198, 206-
    207
  chlorambucil, 82-84, 88
  daunomycin, 16, 56, 67
  GYK-DTPA, 101-107, 110-116
  HRP, 188, 190, 197-198
  idarubicin, 78-80, 82, 87-88
  methotrexate (MTX), 56-62, 67,
    81-82
  N-acetyl-melphalan, 82-85
  ricin, 42, 85-87, 88, 90-92
  toxicity, 15-16
Immunofluorescence testing, 220-
    221, 227
Immunomagnetic depletion, 139-
    141, 145-147
Immunometric assay (see Radioim-
    munoassay)
Immunoreactivity of GYK-DTPA
    antibody, 103-106
Immunoscintigraphy (see Radioim-
    munoscintigraphy)
Immunotherapy, 16-23, 110-116
  anti-idiotypic, 17, 20-23
  212Bi, 110-116
  131I, 13, 56, 61-62
  111In, 56, 103-104, 106-108,
    110-111, 114-115
  p175, 21-22
  recombinant live virus, 17-20
  vp97, 18-20
  90Y, 110-116

[Immunotherapy]
  yttrium, 110-116
Immunotoxins
  cytotoxicity activity, 46-47, 57-59,
    63-64
  enhancer HSA-monensin, 46-47,
    50-51
  Fab, 46-48
  F(ab)'2, 46-47, 92-93
  ricin A chain, 7, 15, 41-46, 50,
    67-69
  ricin B chain, 42, 139
  T101, 44, 46-49,
111In (see Indium-111)
Indium-111, 56, 103-104, 106-108,
    110-111, 114-115
Interferon, 10, 16
Iodine-125, 55, 61, 120-125, 130
Iodine-131, 13, 56, 56-62
Isoelectric focusing (IEF), 102

L

L6, 12-13, 16
Latex particles (see Protein-coated
    latex particles)
Latex spheres, 157-168 (see also
    Site-specific covalent coupling)
Leukemia cell lines, 18-20, 120-132,
    137-139, 142-147
  T-cell, 137-139, 143-144
  B-ALL, 137-139, 143-144
  B-CLL, 42, 48-51
  BL, 143-146
  B-lymphoma, 7-8, 11
  Ly-2.1, 75
Lymphocytic leukemia (B-CLL) (see
    Leukemia cell lines)

M

Magnetic tape chromium dioxide,
    201-215
Melanoma cells, 3-8
Methotrexate (MTX), 56-62, 67, 81-
    82

[Methotrexate (MTX)]
  conjugation to HSA, 57-59, 61
  conjugation to 791T/36, 57-62,
    67-69
  cytotoxicity of, 57-59
MG-21, 9, 21
Monoclonal antibodies (MAb) (*see
    also* specific antibodies)
  amino acids linkage, 43-46
  anti-CD5 T101, 44, 46-48
  anti-CFR, 225
  anti-CMV, 171, 174-175
  anti-p97, 3-7, 18
  anti-PIV, 176-179
  anti-Thy 1.2, 45, 50-51
  B72.3, 103-104, 106-107, 113-
    116
  bone marrow purging, 139, 145,
    147
  crosslinking of, 121-123, 128-129
  disulfide bridge, 42-43, 62-64
  2H7, 12-13
  L6, 12-13, 16
  Ly-2.1, 75
  MG-21, 9, 21
  R9.75, 102-104, 109
  site specific, 101, 103-106, 108-
    109, 155-184
  thioether bridge, 43-44
  6.10, 21-22
  48.7, 6
  96.5, 5-6
  791T/36, 54-69
  V1-10 mAb, 120-132
Murine thymoma, 75, 86, 90

N

N-acetyl-melphalan, 82-85
  drug-antibody conjugation, 82-84
96.5, 5-6
N-succinimidyl-3-(2-pyridyldithio)
    (SPDP), 42-43, 85, 121, 123-
    124, 130, 132
  crosslinking with, 121-123

O

Ovarian carcinomas, 54-56
Oxidation of antibody carbohydrate,
    161-162, 174

P

P97, 3-7, 18-20
  in vitro localization of anti-p97,
    5-6
  molecular nature, 4
  specificity, 3
  therapeutic approaches to, 6-7
  transfection of mouse melanomas,
    5
  transferrin, relation to, 4
P175, 21-22
PAGE (*see* Polyacrylamide gel
    electrophoresis)
Pharmacokinetic studies, 65-66
Polyacrylamide gel electrophoresis
    (PAGE), 183
Protein-coated latex particles (CLP),
    218-228
  agglutination, 218, 220, 225-226,
    228
  binding with CFR, 221-226, 228
  localization of, 221-223, 228

R

R9.75, 102-104, 109
Radioimmunoassay (RIA), 61-62,
    169-175, 201-215
  enzyme immunometric assay
    (EIA), 187-188
Radioimmunoscinitigraphy, 61-62,
    107-110
Radioimmunotherapy (*see* Immuno-
    therapy)
Radiolabeled MAb, 13-14
Renal cell carcinoma, 23
RIA (*see* radioimmunoassay)

Ricin
   drug-antibody conjugation, 85-87,
     88, 90-92
   toxicity, 85
Ricin A chain(RIA), 7, 15, 41-46,
   50, 62-69
   conjugation to 791T/36, 62-69
Ricin B chain, 42, 139

S

SDS-PAGE (*see* Sodium dodecylsulfate (SDS)-polyacrylamide gel
   electrophoresis)
Site-specific covalent coupling, 155-
   185 (*see also* Monoclonal antibodies)
  of glycoprotein via:
   latex spheres, 157-168
    antimated, 158
    carboxylated, 157
    fetuin, 165
    magnetic, 166
    nitrocellulose strips, 168-169
    nylon strips, 169
    polystyrene plates, 168
   6.10, 21-22
Sodium dodecylsulfate (SDS)poly-
   acrylamide gel electrophoresis
   (SDS-PAGE), 55-56, 121-123,
   130, 132
SPDP (*see* N-succinimidyl-3(2-pyri-
   dyldithio))

T

791T/36, 54-69
   conjugation to methotrexate, 56-
    62, 67-69
   conjugation to ricin A chain, 62-69
   HSA (human serum albumin),
    56-62, 67-69
   131I antibody conjugates, 56, 60-
    62

[791T/36]
   localization of, 56
T101, 44, 46-49
T cells, 16-18, 20, 44, 48, 50, 137-
   138, 144
Target cell lines (*see also* Leukemia
   cell lines)
   CEM, 44, 47
   COLO 205 (colon), 75-94
   HT29 (colon), 75-94
   K562 (human myelogenous leu-
    kemia), 120-132
   LS174T (colon), 114-115
   P3NSI (murine myeloma), 54
   T2, 52
   791T (osteogenic sarcoma), 54,
    57-59, 63-65
Thy 1.2, 50
TNF (*see* Tumor necrosis factor)
Transferrin, 4
Tumor heterogeneity, 92-93
Tumor models, murine thymoma,
   75, 86, 90
Tumor necrosis factor (TNF), 88-89

V

V1-10 mAb:
   conjugated to C3b, 120-132
   crosslinked
    using glutaraldehyde, 121-123
    using SPDP, 121-123
Vaccines, tumor (*see* Immunotherapy)
vp97, 18-20

X Y Z

xenograph, 15, 59-61, 64-67, 106-
   108, 114-115
90Y (*see* Yttrium-90)
Yttrium-90, 110-116